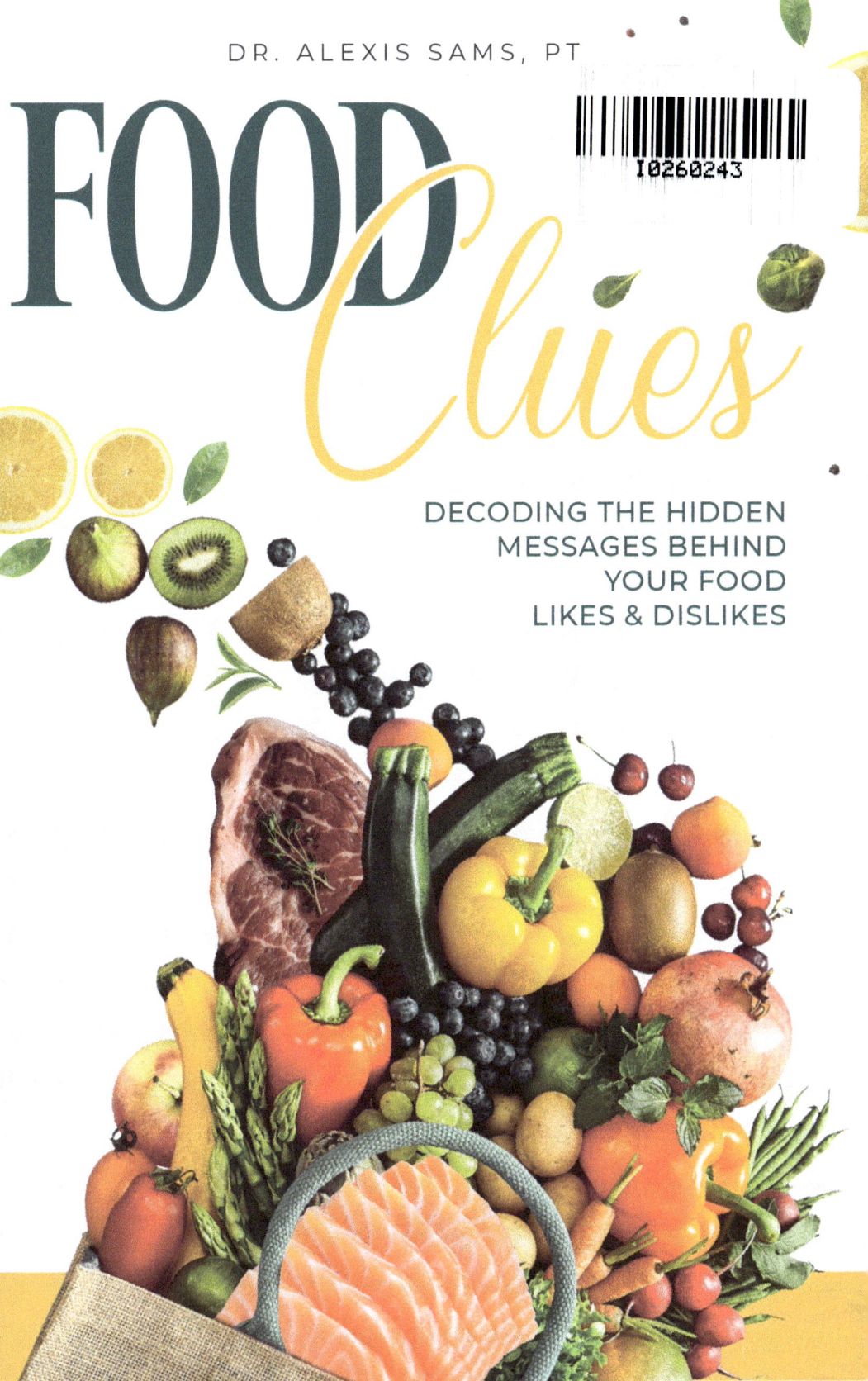

DR. ALEXIS SAMS, PT

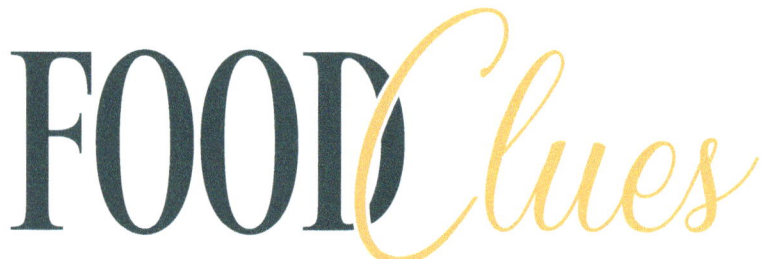

DECODING THE HIDDEN MESSAGES
BEHIND YOUR FOOD LIKES AND DISLIKES

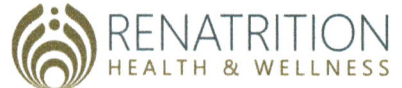

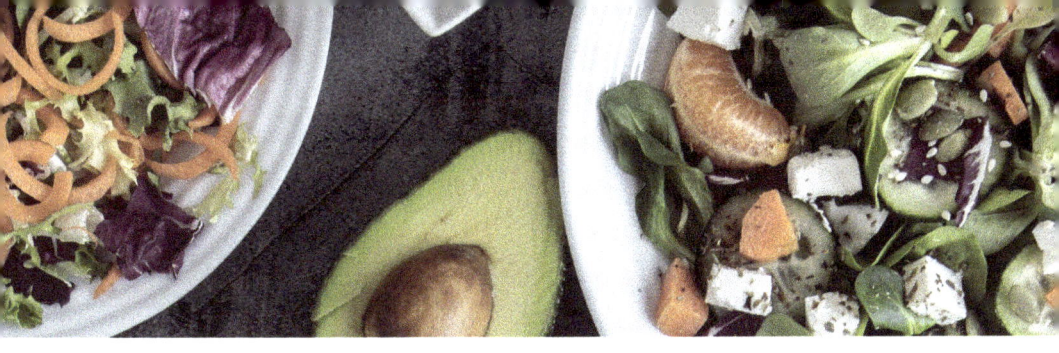

MEDICAL DISCLAIMER

The information provided in this book, "Food Clues: Decoding the Hidden Messages Behind Your Food Likes and Dislikes," is for educational purposes only. It is not intended as a substitute for professional medical advice, diagnosis, or treatment. Always seek the advice of your physician or another qualified health provider with any questions you may have regarding a medical condition. Never disregard professional medical advice or delay seeking it because of something you have read in this book.

The author, Dr. Alexis Sams, PT is not a medical physician. The content of this book is based on her personal experiences, research, and professional knowledge as a holistic physical therapist and functional medicine specialist. The information provided here should not be considered as medical advice or a diagnosis. Individual health circumstances vary, and readers should consult with a qualified healthcare professional for personalized advice regarding their specific situation.

The author and publisher disclaim responsibility for any adverse effects resulting directly or indirectly from the information presented in this book. The reader assumes full responsibility for consulting a qualified healthcare professional regarding health conditions, and the author and publisher are not liable for any outcomes resulting from the use of information provided in this book.

ISBN: 979-8-9897094-0-3

DEDICATION

I dedicate this book to all who have struggled with prolonged symptoms and disease, not knowing that foods can provide clues and be the missing link to their healing . . .

. . . and to me for having the courage to tell you.

"My wish is to give the kind of truth to people that will help them change their minds. When that happens, I'll be the best that I can be...."

—Tina Turner

Table of Contents

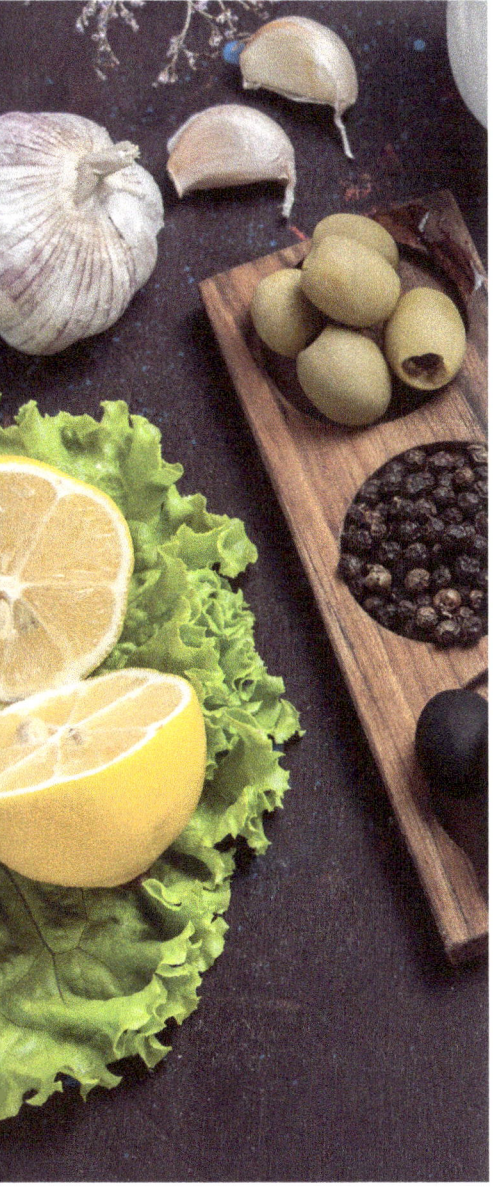

Preface	6
Introduction	8
Inspiration	9
About the book & how to use it	11

Common Food Avoidances

Avocado	16
Banana	20
Beans	24
Blue Cheese	26
Breastmilk	28
Carrots	30
Celery	32
Cilantro	34
Coconut	36
Cucumbers	40
Eggs	42
Garlic	46
Gluten	49
Kiwi	54
Lemon	56
Lettuce	60
Melons	64
Milk	66
Mushrooms	70
Mustard	74
Nuts	78
Onions	82
Peanuts	86
Peas	90

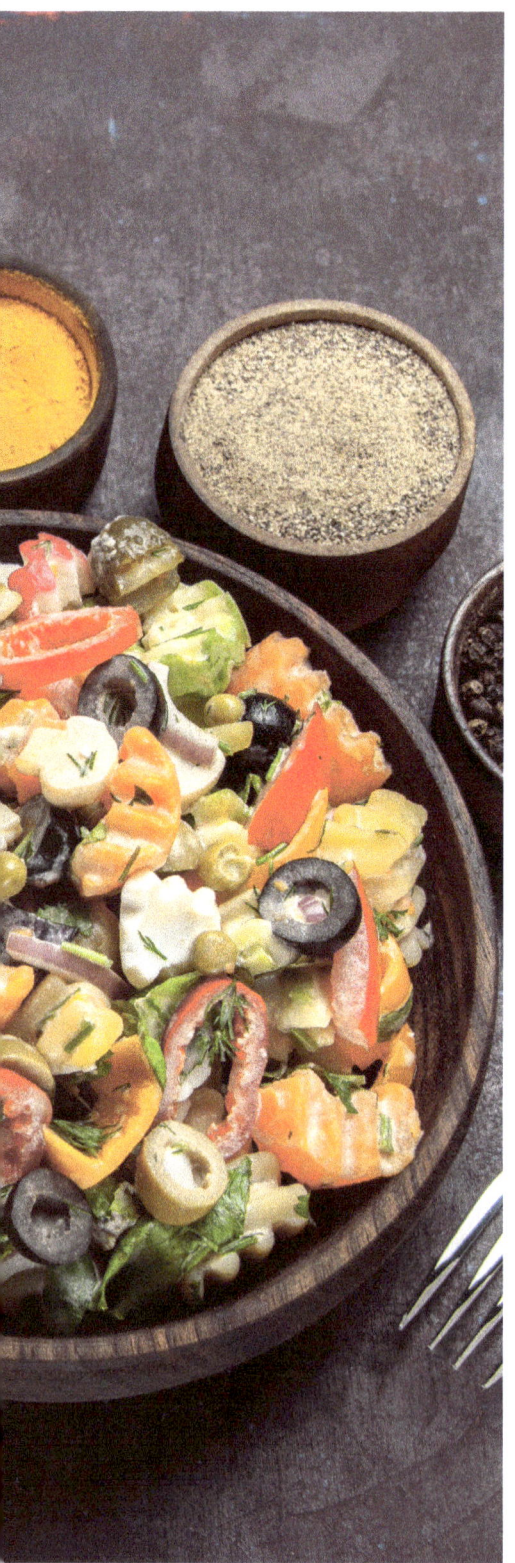

Pepper & Spices	92
Pineapple	96
Salmon & Other Fish	98
Sesame	102
Shrimp & Other Shellfish	106
Soy	110
Steak	112
Strawberries	116
Tomatoes	120
Vinegar	124
Wheat	126

Cravings and habits — 129

What does it all mean? — 134

Fundamentals of healing — 137

   Understanding root causes
   How does illness occur?
   How does the body prioritize healing?
   Using food as clues vs. food as medicine

Starting your healing journey — 147

Finding a wellness practitioner
   A quick overview of the Renatrition Healing Framework
   Want to work with me?

Final thoughts — 154

Add-ons — 156

The truth about food allergies
   Client success stories
   Frequently Asked Questions

About Dr. Alexis — 171

Acknowledgments — 174

References — 176

PREFACE

My husband used to be obsessed with mustard. It had to go on every sandwich. He would choose our dinner meals based on how many things he could put mustard on. It would be the base of every marinade. He dipped his french fries in mustard instead of ketchup. The cravings were insane. Weird, right?

A couple I knew joked about their sneak-away dates to Chik-fil-A. They would have their getaways whenever their daughter stayed with her grandparents. Why? Well, poor thing had a peanut allergy, and if you didn't know, Chik-fil-A fries their chicken in peanut oil. So they had to be super sneaky about their special rendezvous. But it's not just them. Everywhere I go, people seem to be talking about their food allergies, sensitivities or cravings. Gluten, soy, dairy, sugar and salt—the list never ends!

I have so many stories of hearing people talk about how their life is affected by the foods they can't eat or the ones they incessantly crave. Many have found ways to manage and keep a relatively happy lifestyle. Others remain frustrated and wish there was more that they could do to prevent a possible digestive attack or flare up of a condition because of a

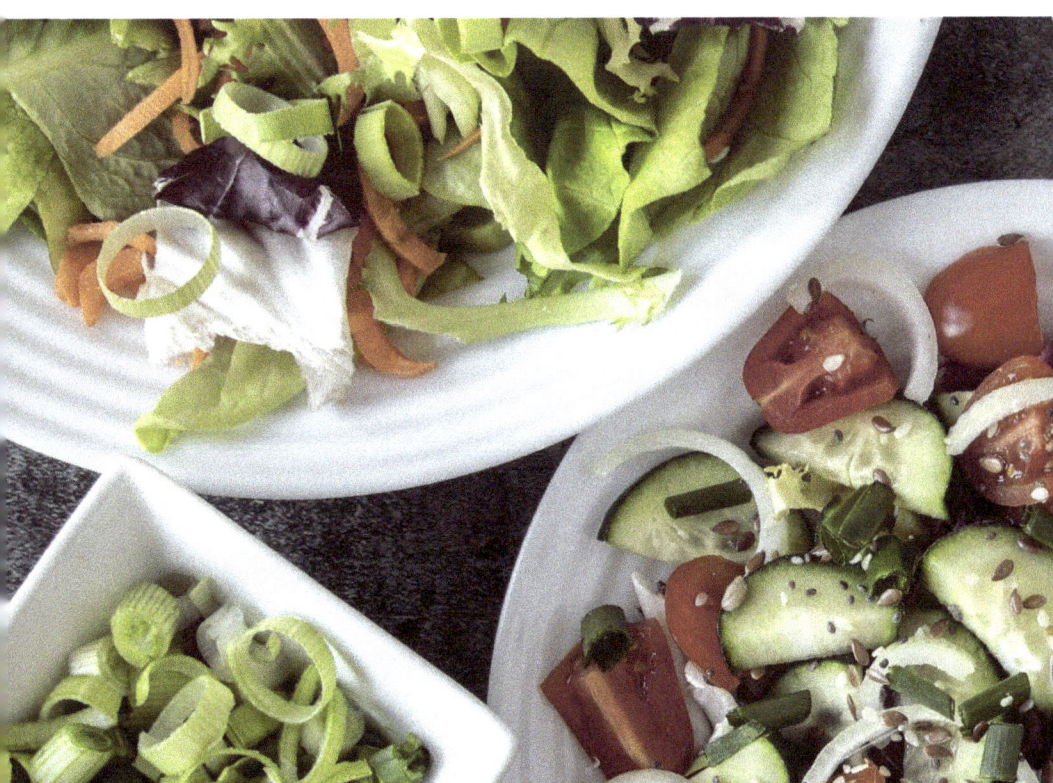

food they overlooked during a meal.

I've built a career from being unconventional, going against the grain, and straying from popular opinion, and this book is no different. The connections between our food choices and our health extend beyond just personal preferences; they serve as valuable clues in unraveling the mysteries behind persistent symptoms and conditions that prove challenging to control or eliminate. I am going to show you that there is the possibility of freedom from having to worry about how your next meal may affect your day, week, or life.

If you or someone you know struggles to enjoy life because of the foods they hate, or the foods they hate to love, this book is the first step to food freedom.

· ·

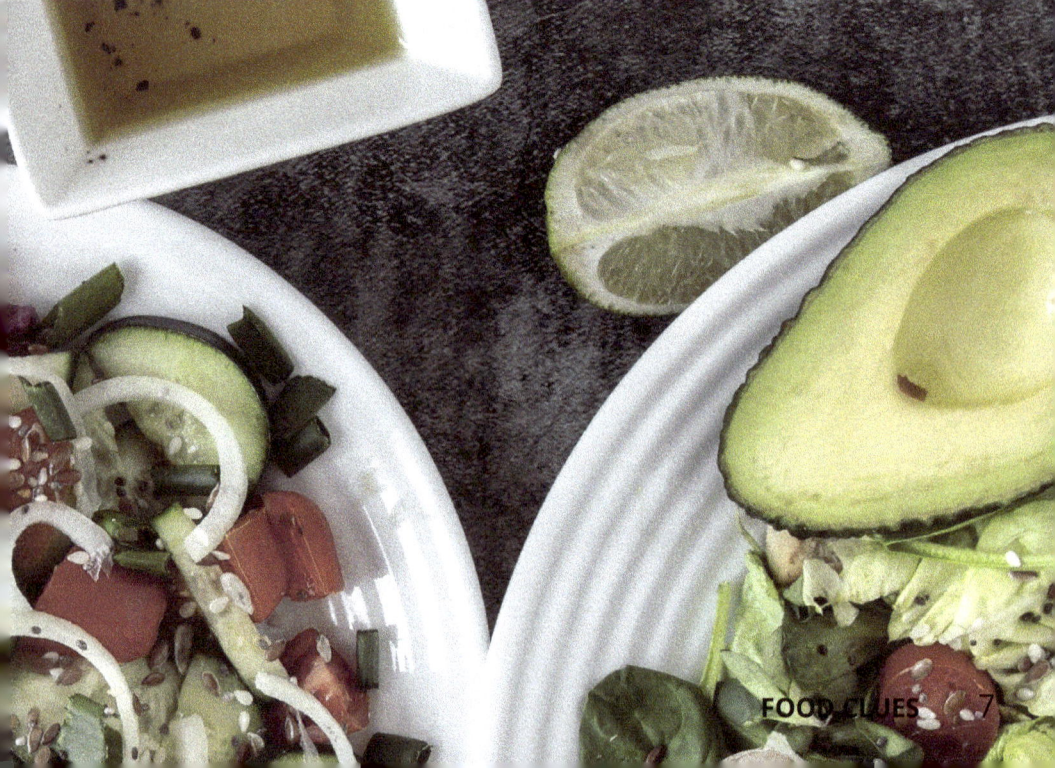

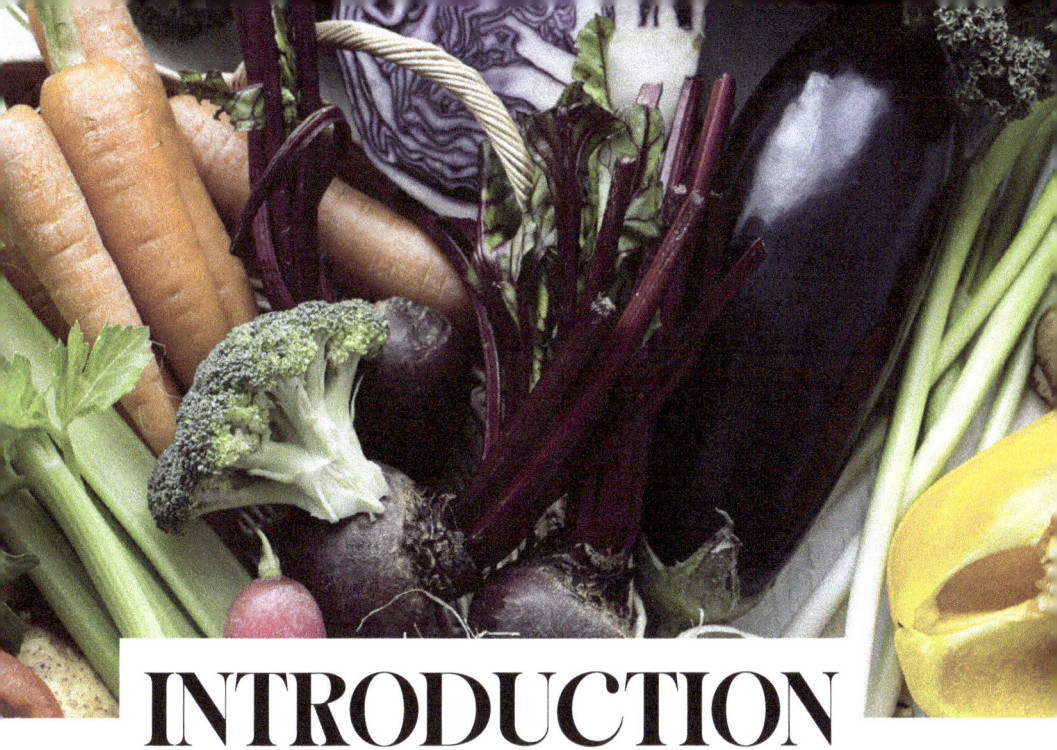

INTRODUCTION

· ·

Have you ever wondered why your taste buds crave certain foods while others leave you cringing? Why you have an odd craving for carrots, while the scent of cilantro can instantly ruin a dish for you? Why some foods make you gassy, give you belly pain, or go right through you? The world of food is full of intriguing mysteries, but within it lies the keys to living a healthier life.

Welcome to Food Clues: Decoding the Hidden Messages Behind Your Food Likes and Dislikes. In this groundbreaking book, you can explore the profound connection between your food preferences and your health. By understanding the hidden messages within your likes and dislikes - including everything from general avoidances to actual sensitivities, reactions, and formal allergies - you can uncover vital clues about the status of your body systems and begin a journey of knowledge and healing to help you live your best life..

Food is an integral part of our existence. It sustains us, nourishes us, and has a profound impact on our overall well-being. Yet many of us go through life without truly understanding the powerful relationship between the foods we consume and the intricate workings of our bodies. We may dismiss our food likes and dislikes as mere matters of personal preference or attribute them to family genetics, unaware of the valuable insights they hold.

But what if I told you that your food preferences are more than just whimsical cravings or dislikes? What if I revealed that they are powerful clues, guiding us toward a path of optimal health and vitality? It is through these food clues that you can unlock the secrets to understanding and addressing the symptoms and issues that keep you from living a happier and healthier life.

Our bodies are remarkably intricate systems, interconnected and delicately balanced. Every cell, organ, and body system relies on a complex dance of nutrients and biological processes to function optimally. When this delicate balance is disrupted, it can manifest as a wide range of symptoms and health issues, from fatigue and mental imbalances to digestive disorders and other system conditions.

By embracing the concept of food as health clues, you empower yourself to take control of your health and well-being. By understanding the hidden messages within your food likes and dislikes, you can identify dietary patterns that may be contributing to your health challenges and make informed choices to support your healing journey.

It is my hope that Food Clues serves as a guide and a source of inspiration for you to embark on a transformative journey toward optimal health. Get ready to discover the hidden messages behind your food likes and dislikes.

Dr. Alexis Sams, PT

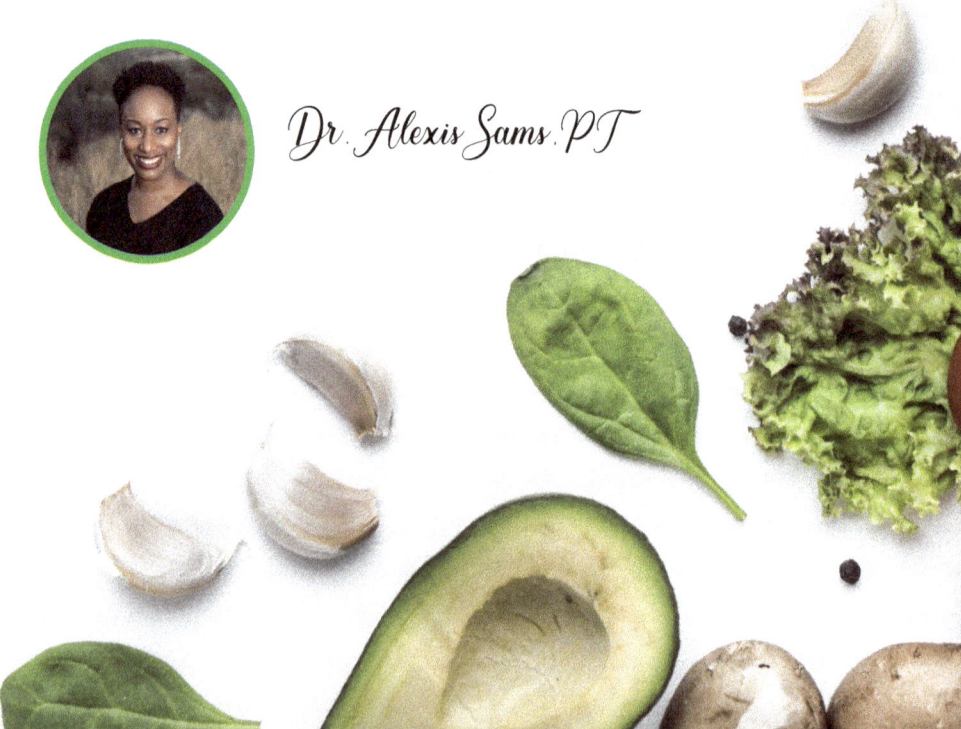

Inspiration
So why did I decide to write Food Clues?

In short, to help more people than I can reach in a workweek.

Everyone has a story of how the 2020 Covid pandemic changed their life, and this is mine. If you know me, then you know that I am the owner of AZ Dance Medicine Specialists in Phoenix, Arizona, a specialty clinic that focuses on rehabilitation and performance enhancement for dancers and other artists. During the pandemic, dance facilities and art venues were considered non-essential and were shut down, crippling my business almost to the point of closing. However, many clients and their friends and families knew that my work with dancers included functional medicine and holistic care, and many of them reached out asking for help to boost their immunity to protect them from the virus. Over the year, I gained more and more clients, and by 2021 I expanded to open a clinic fully focused on functional medicine and holistic health, Renatrition Health and Wellness.

As my clientele at Renatrition grew, I began to notice patterns. Potential clients with diagnosed conditions almost always had some type of food sensitivity or allergy included in their medical history. Then I remembered from my functional medicine training that certain foods related to certain organ dysfunctions, like how hating cilantro correlated to poor liver detox and that gluten sensitivity related to poor protein digestion in the intestines. So I began to wonder if other foods provided similar clues to organ or system functions. Turns out, they do!

I added a food preference assessment to my client intake form, and before clients even showed up for their first session, I had an idea of which organs and systems were in trouble and even got a few ideas on how they had developed issues. The clues I gained from food preferences has become my number one diagnostic tool for faster and more effective treatment and recovery for my clients. As my success with resolving clients' symptoms grew, I knew I needed to help more people learn about the connections between food preferences and what they could mean for their health and performance. This is my solution, a simple guide to help you gain more insight into your personal health from a perspective that very few wellness practitioners are talking about.

About the Book
& How to use it

This book isn't just about reading it from cover to cover; it's a dynamic resource designed to guide you through your body's relationship with food. Here, I'll walk you through how to navigate Food Clues to get the most out of it.

Understanding the journey ahead:

Within the pages of Food Clues, you'll embark on a journey of self-discovery and empowerment. This book was created to support you through various scenarios. Whether you're facing a food that doesn't agree with you or offering a helping hand to a friend or loved one, this book is your trusty companion.

The layout at a glance:

I've meticulously created a range of topics to provide you with a holistic understanding of the intricate dance between your body, your food choices, and your well-being. Feel free to skip around and read the sections that most interest you. Start reading about the foods that affect you or your friends and family the most, read about how I treat my clients, or check out my thoughts on common myths about food allergies.

Decoding food relationships:

Food Clues delivers detailed profiles for 35 commonly avoided foods. Each profile not only outlines the food's nutritional value but also sheds light on the typical responses that lead to avoidance. In the 'Food Clue Category' section, I delve into the underlying issues within the body that drive these avoidances. And, in the 'Health Concerns' section, you'll find common conditions often linked to the specific food clue category behind the avoidance.

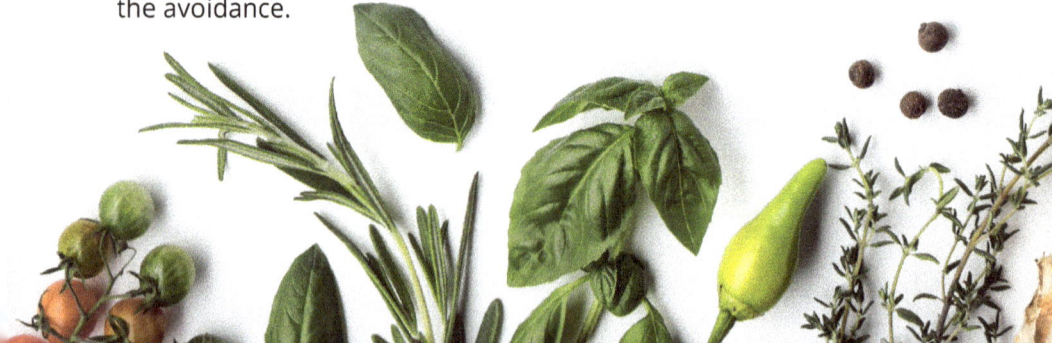

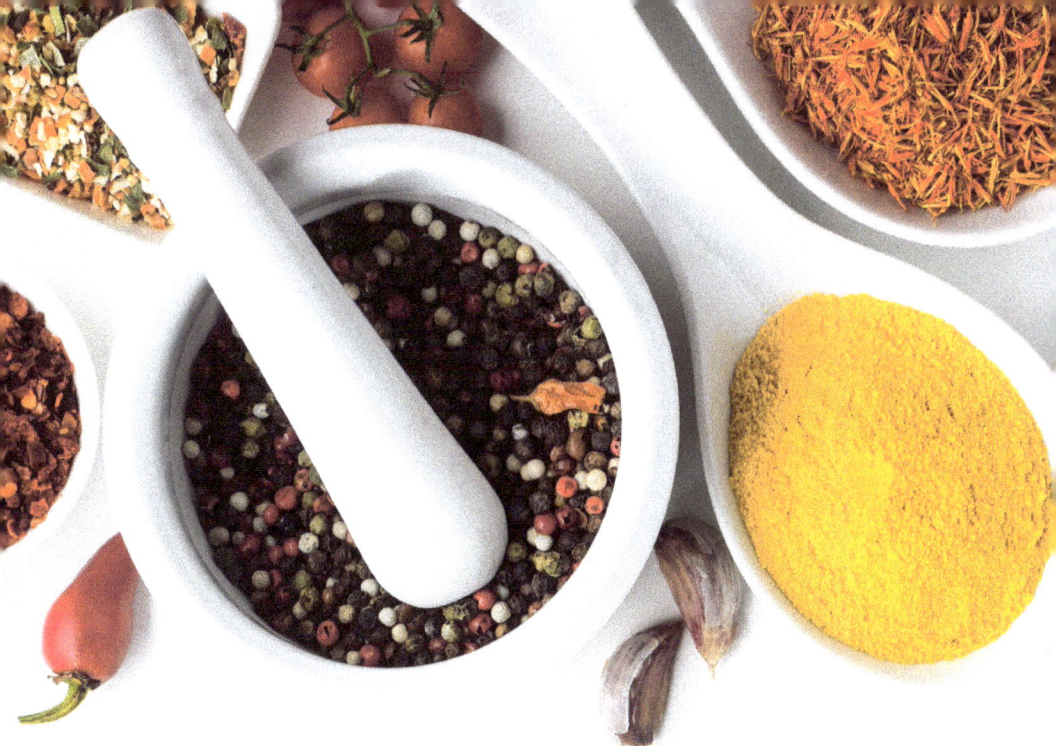

Unraveling cravings and patterns:

The exploration doesn't stop there. I also include the meaning behind ten common food cravings, gaining insights into their implications for your health. Further, I uncover the significance of five distinct food eating patterns or habits, enhancing your comprehension of your dietary inclinations.

Guiding you on the healing path:

Venture deeper into the heart of the book, where I offer an overview of the illness spectrum. This section unveils the body's intricate responses to illness, shining a light on how it prioritizes healing and recovery. Following this, I introduce my personal treatment framework, designed to put you on the fastest, safest track to transformative results. This framework is the culmination of years of dedication, research, and experience.

Inspiring stories and clarifications:

Within these pages, you'll also find captivating client success stories that affirm the potency of decoding food clues in identifying and addressing the root causes of health challenges.

Embracing the content:

As you immerse yourself in this wealth of knowledge, remember that Food Clues is a piece of a larger puzzle. While it draws from my practical experience and studies, it isn't exhaustive. Your unique journey encompasses a myriad of factors beyond these pages.

What food clues is and isn't:

It's important to clarify the intention of Food Clues. This book doesn't provide a definitive list of meanings or solutions for food likes and dislikes. Nor does it replace the guidance of qualified health professionals. The insights shared here are part of your puzzle, not an exclusive solution.

A collaborative approach:

While the content is invaluable, it's not a substitute for medical care and provides no diagnosis for any medical condition. The foods listed reflect my learning journey—they're not mandates, just tools for understanding. They do not advocate for specific dietary choices or restrictions, nor do they pass judgment on any dietary preferences. My purpose is to provide understanding and support, not to prescribe a rigid dietary approach.

With this understanding, dive into Food Clues as your compass for decoding your relationship with food. May it empower you to make informed choices, offering insights for yourself and those around you. Together, let's embark on this transformative voyage of self-discovery, healing, and renewed well-being.

• •

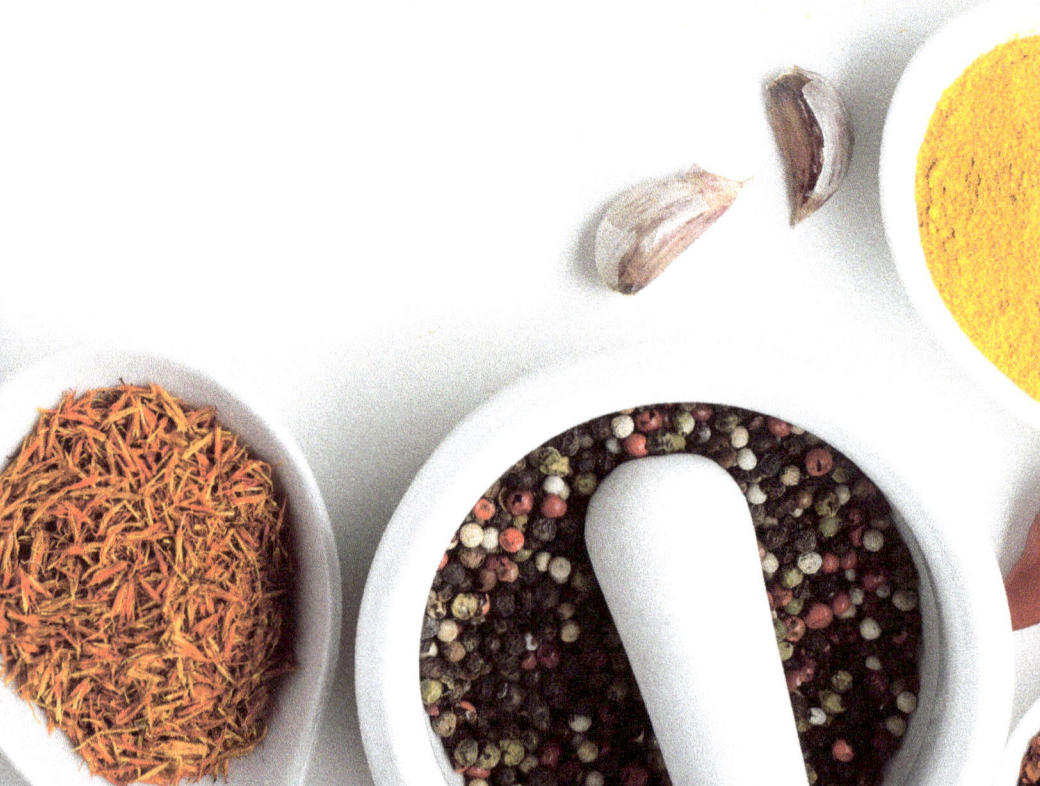

> "TELL ME WHAT YOU EAT, AND I WILL TELL YOU WHO YOU ARE."
>
> - Jean Anthelme Brillat-Savarin,
> French lawyer and gastronome

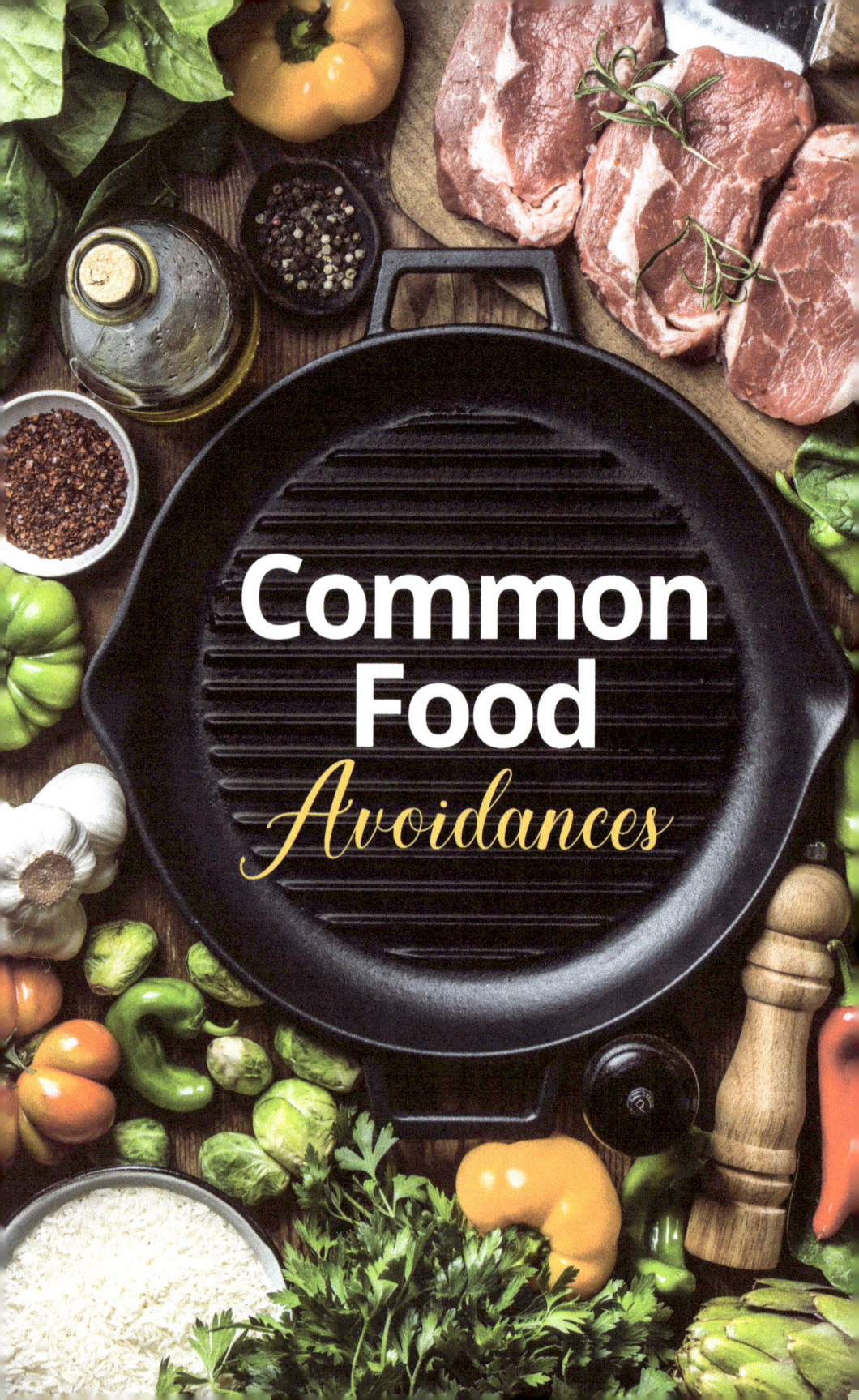

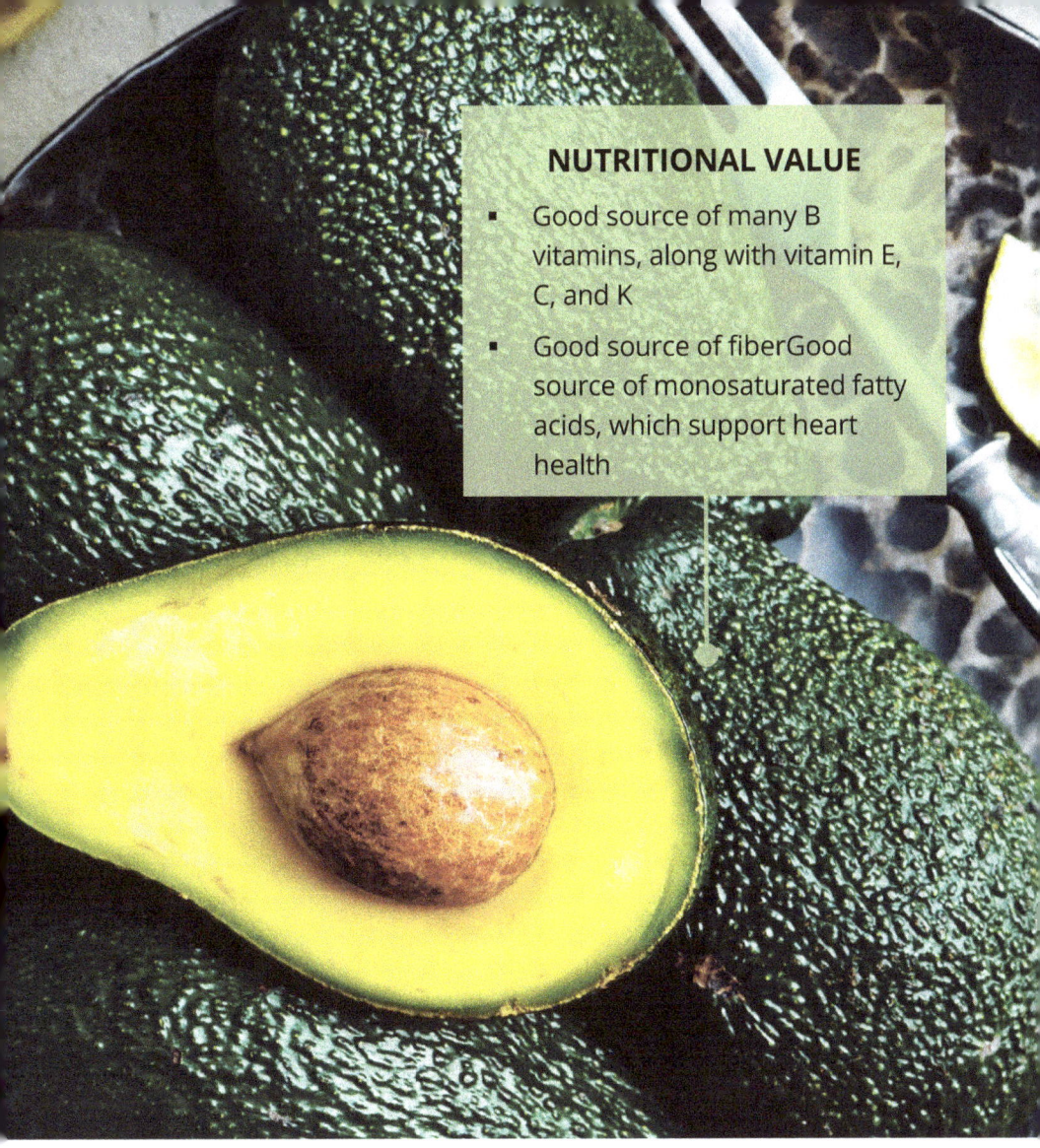

NUTRITIONAL VALUE

- Good source of many B vitamins, along with vitamin E, C, and K
- Good source of fiberGood source of monosaturated fatty acids, which support heart health

01 Avocado

Common Avoidance *Responses*

- Lip or tongue swelling
- Itchy skin
- Gas, bloating, or nausea

Food Clue *Category*

- Fatty acid imbalance
- Unbalanced gut bacteria levels

Food Clue *Explained*

In many cases, whether you like or hate avocado indicates how balanced your body may be in omega-6 and omega-3 fatty acids. In general, the body likes a 4:1 ratio of omega-6 to omega-3 levels.

Avocado cravings can be a sign of low overall levels of omega-6 and omega-3 fatty acids (the "good fats"), which help manage blood sugar, cholesterol levels, and heart and gut health.

Reactions to avocado usually indicate that the balance between these fatty acids is off, and most often there's an excess of omega-6 fatty acid relative to omega-3 levels.

HEALTH CONCERNS

- Heart disease
- Hormone imbalance
- Adrenal gland dysfunction
- Menstrual cycle dysfunction or conditions including heavy bleeding, missed cycles, endometriosis, and polycystic ovary syndrome (PCOS)
- Emotional and mental health imbalances including anxiety, depression, autism, attention deficit disorder, attention deficit hyperactivity disorder

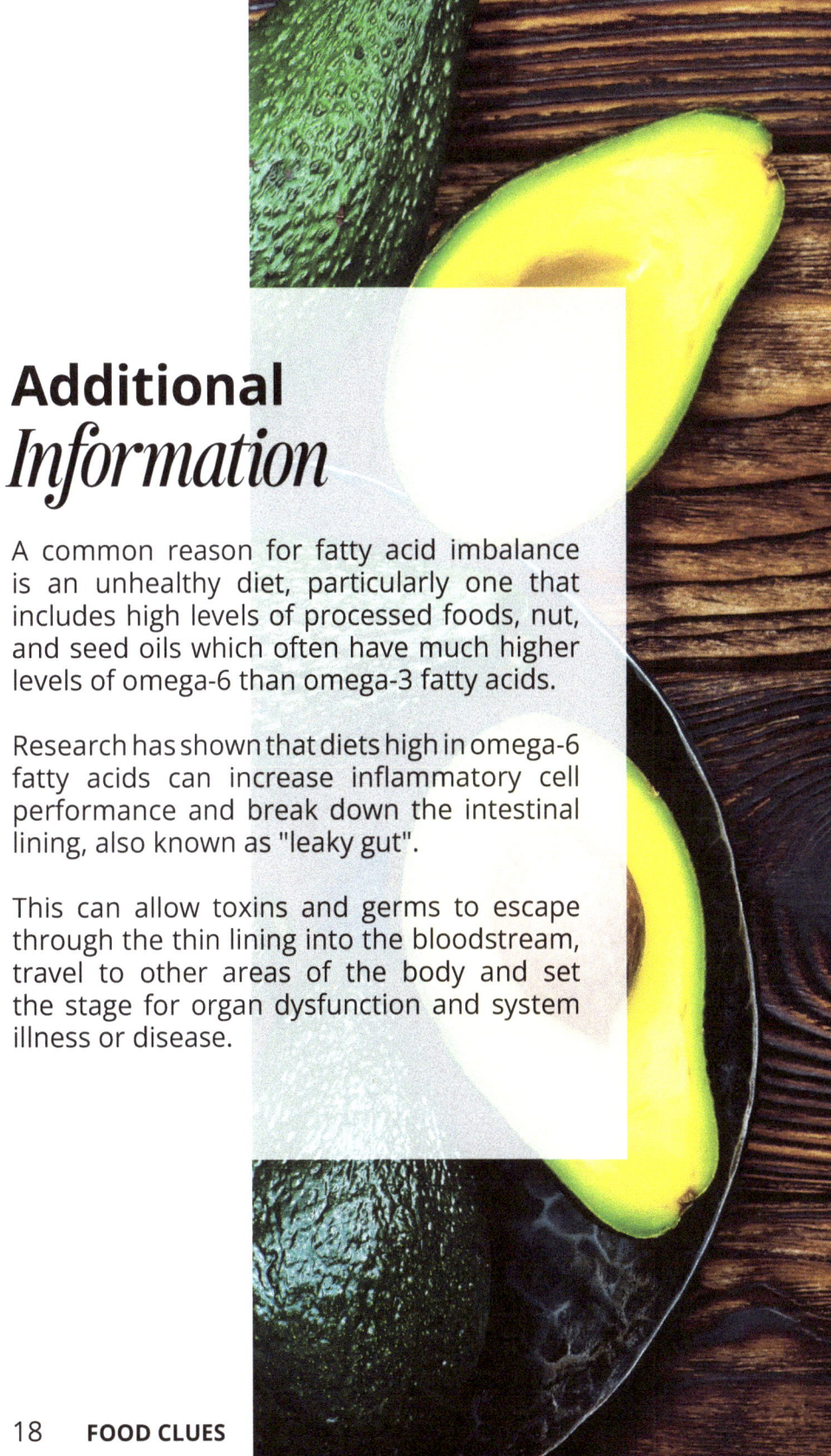

Additional
Information

A common reason for fatty acid imbalance is an unhealthy diet, particularly one that includes high levels of processed foods, nut, and seed oils which often have much higher levels of omega-6 than omega-3 fatty acids.

Research has shown that diets high in omega-6 fatty acids can increase inflammatory cell performance and break down the intestinal lining, also known as "leaky gut".

This can allow toxins and germs to escape through the thin lining into the bloodstream, travel to other areas of the body and set the stage for organ dysfunction and system illness or disease.

"Every food allergy has an underlying cause. Find it, fix it, and enjoy more of life."

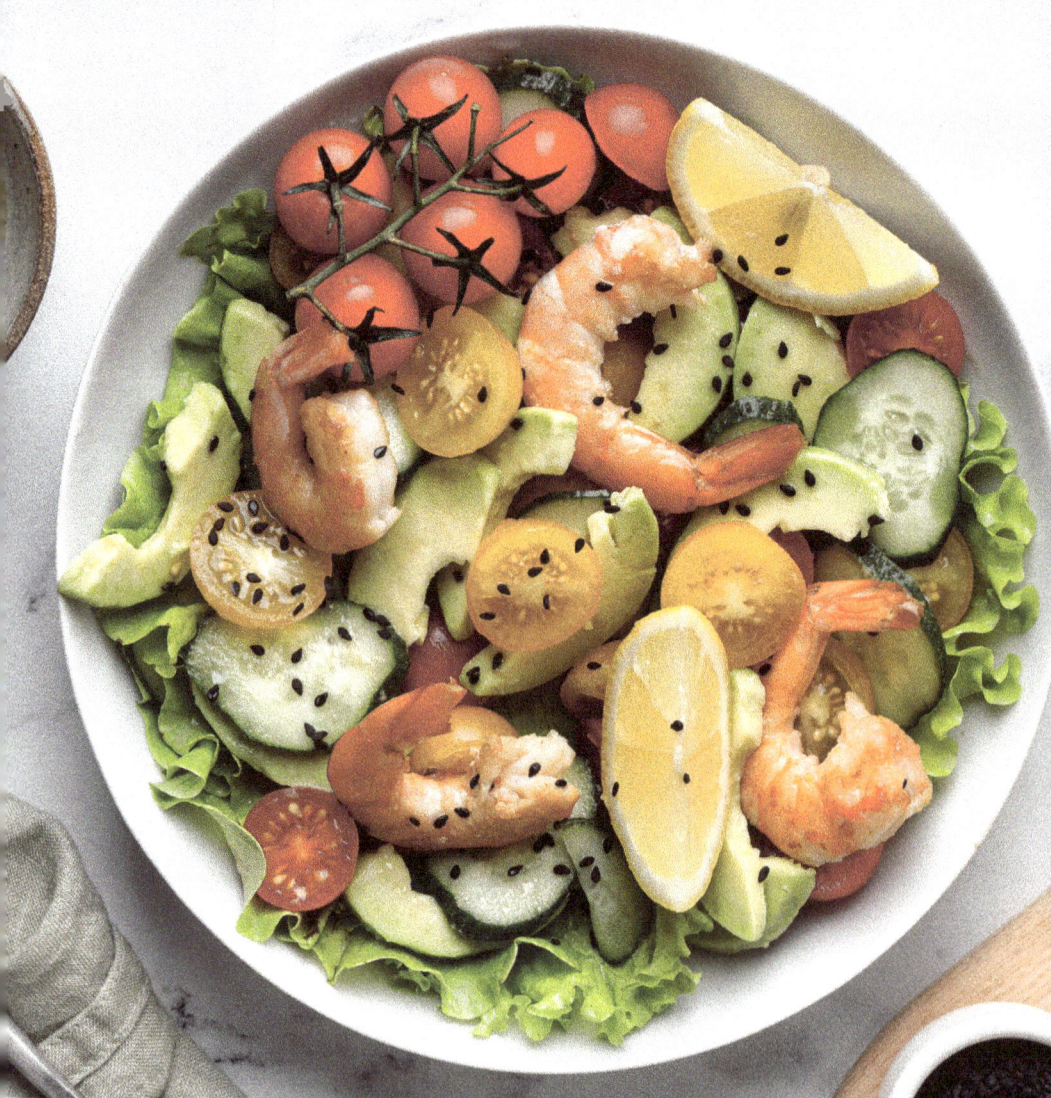

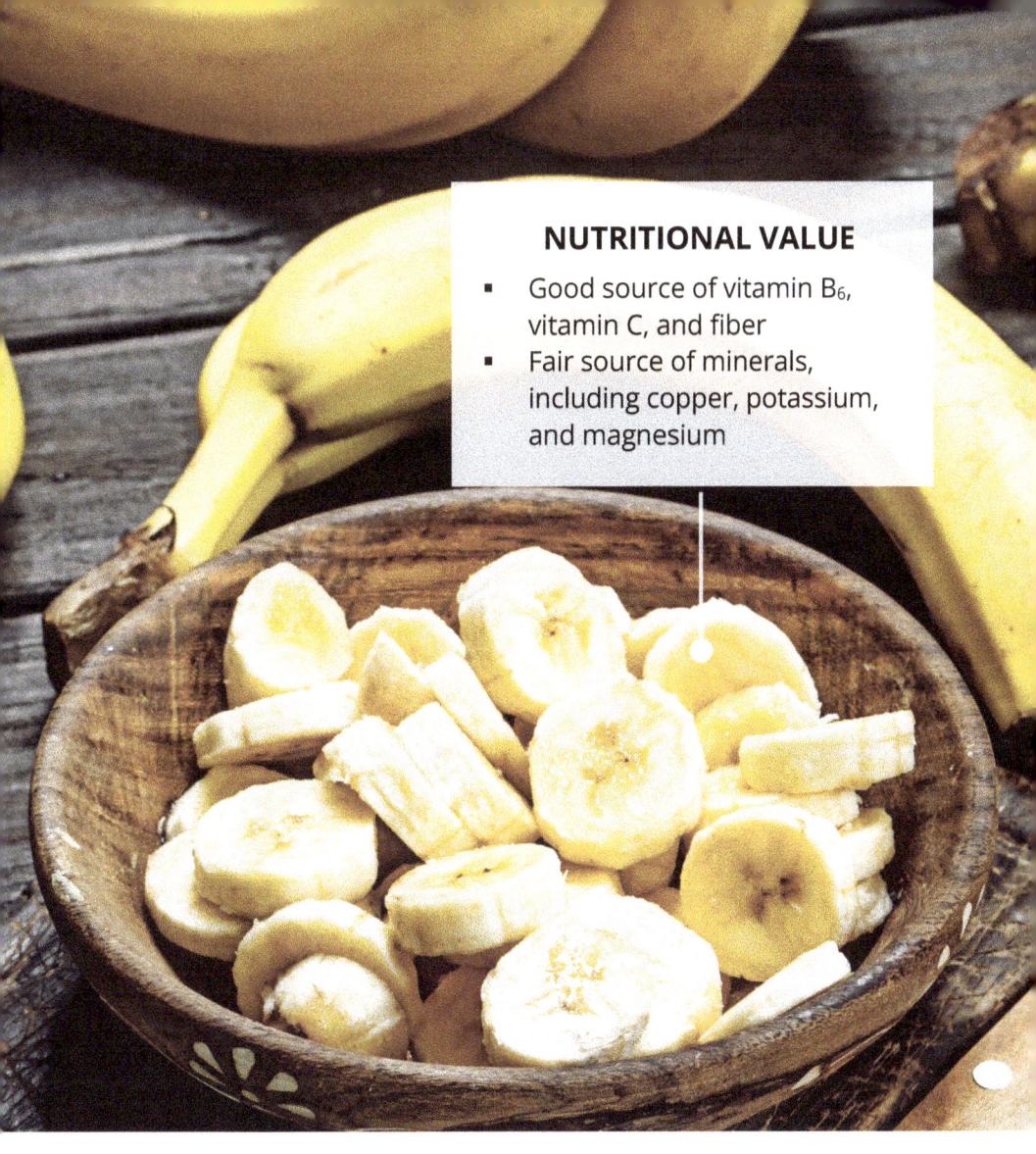

NUTRITIONAL VALUE

- Good source of vitamin B_6, vitamin C, and fiber
- Fair source of minerals, including copper, potassium, and magnesium

02 Banana

Common Avoidance *Responses*

- Lip or tongue swelling
- Itchy skin
- Hives or other skin reactions
- Gas
- Bloating
- Nausea

HEALTH CONCERNS

- Liver or gallbladder dysfunction
- Adrenal gland dysfunction
- Increased risk of infection

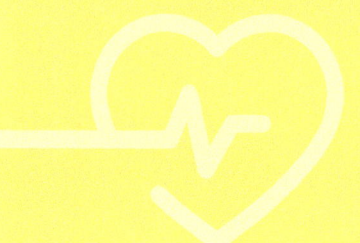

Food Clue *Category*

- Poor nutrient absorption
- Poor protein digestion
- Metal toxicity

Food Clue *Explained*

Reactions to unripe or yellow bananas are mostly related to difficulty digesting a specific protein called *chitinase,* causing more digestive symptoms.

Reactions to more ripe bananas can indicate elevated histamine levels in the body with fewer issues related to protein breakdown. Histamine is released as bananas ripen, as chitinase is broken down, and difficulty managing histamines may result in more skin-related avoidance responses.

Elevated metals in the body or poor use of key minerals can also result in the rejection of bananas, since they have considerable amounts of magnesium, potassium, and copper.

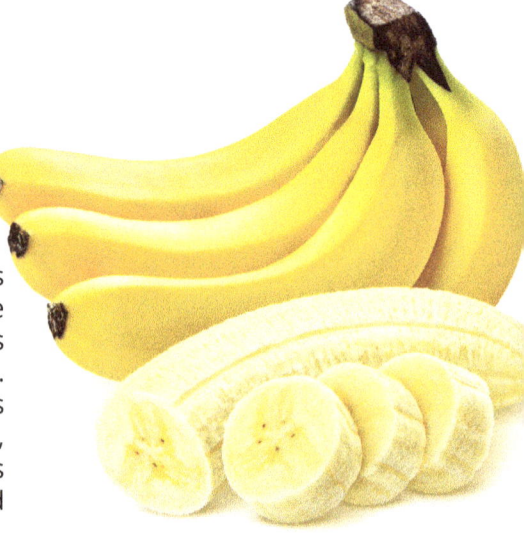

FOOD CLUES   21

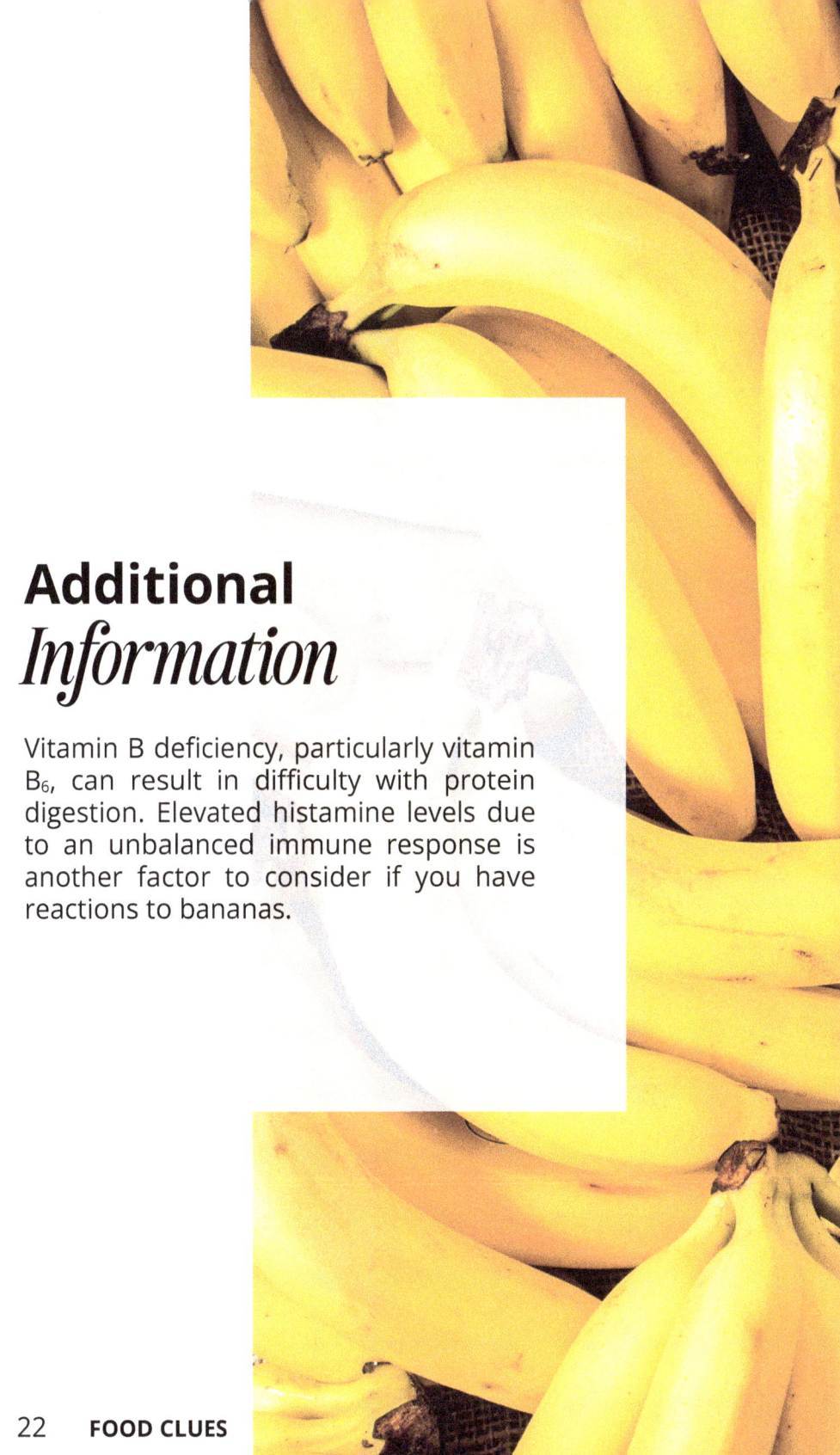

Additional
Information

Vitamin B deficiency, particularly vitamin B_6, can result in difficulty with protein digestion. Elevated histamine levels due to an unbalanced immune response is another factor to consider if you have reactions to bananas.

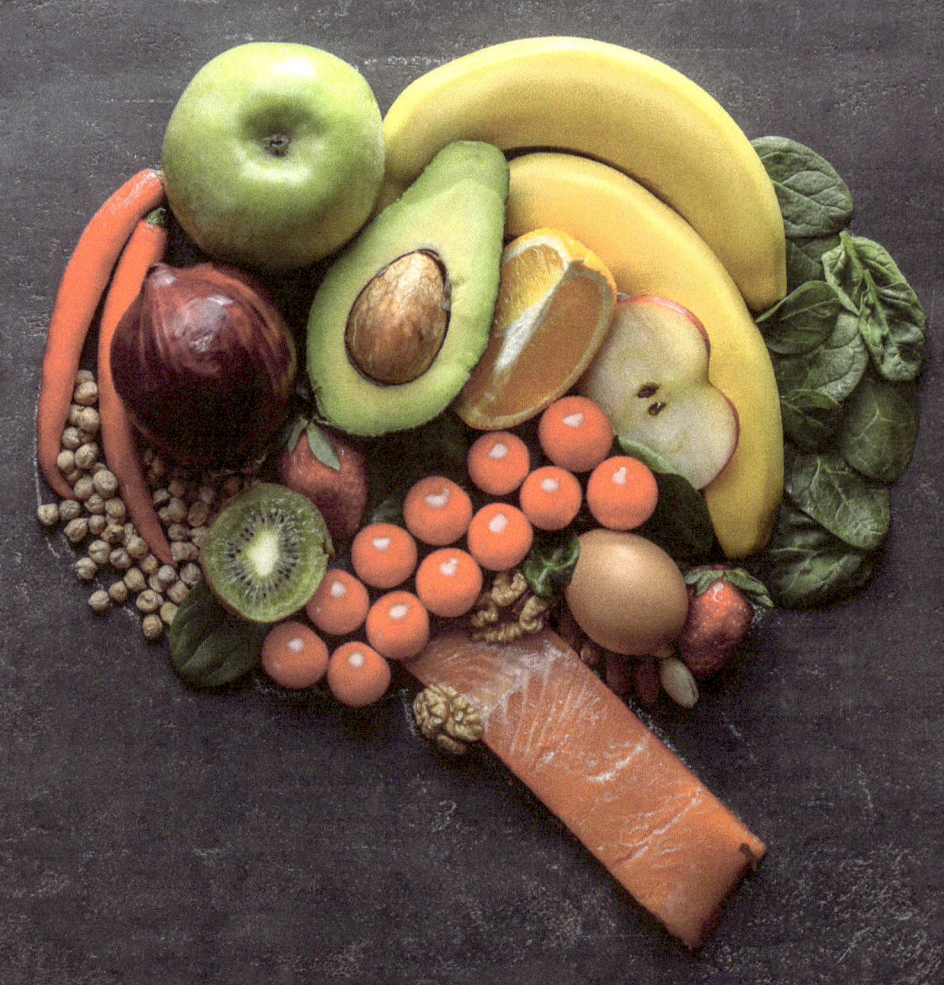

"Anything that affects the gut will always affect the brain."

– Dr. Charles Major

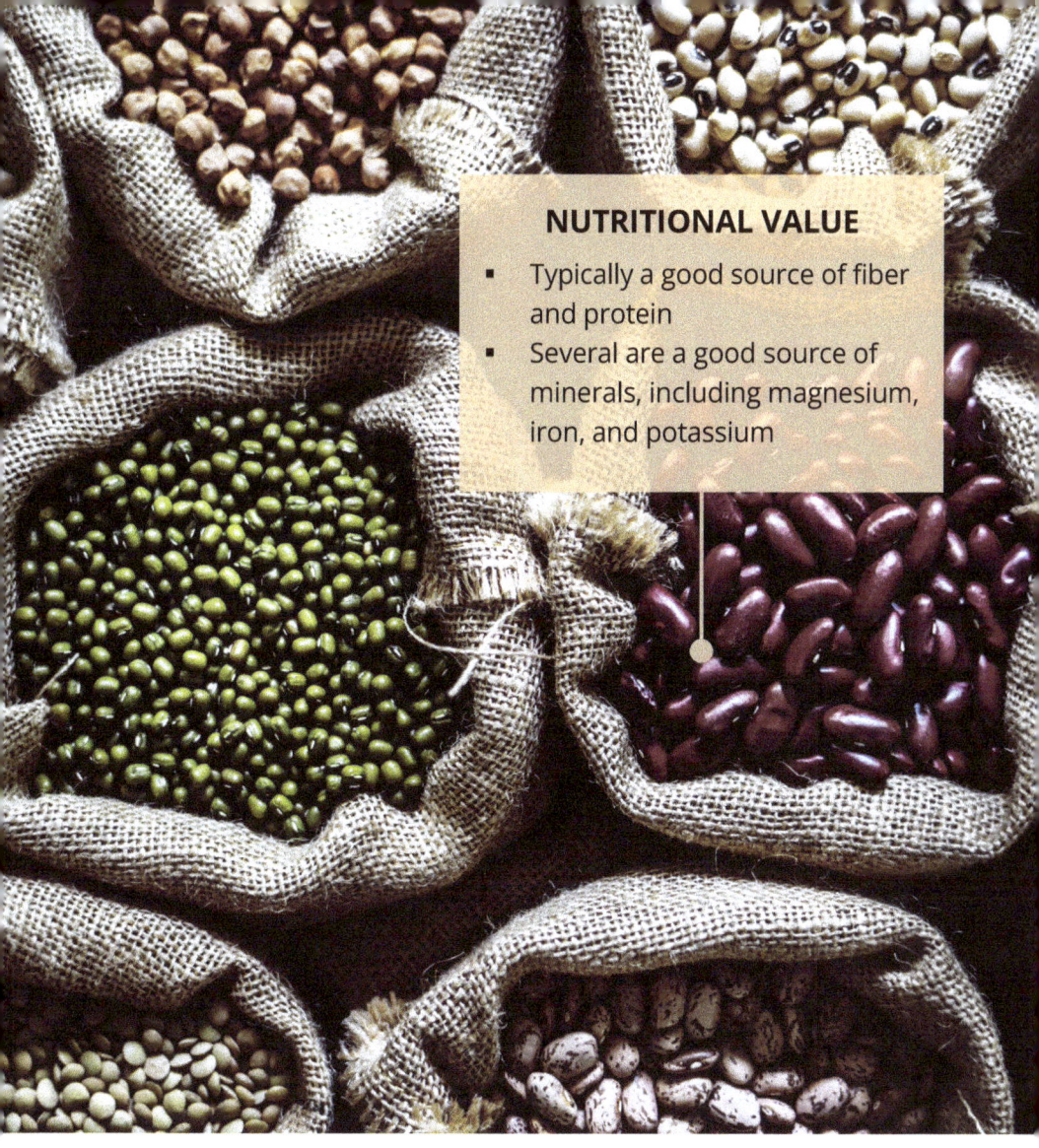

NUTRITIONAL VALUE

- Typically a good source of fiber and protein
- Several are a good source of minerals, including magnesium, iron, and potassium

03 Beans

Common Avoidance *Responses*

- Gas
- Bloating
- Indigestion
- Constipation
- Abdominal pain
- Nausea

Food Clue *Category*

- Poor protein digestion

HEALTH CONCERNS

- Small intestinal bacterial overgrowth (SIBO)
- Digestive conditions including irritable bowel syndrome, Crohn's disease, and celiac disease

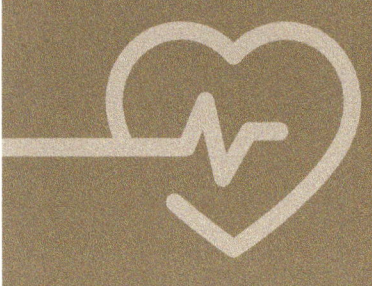

Food Clue *Explained*

Intolerance to beans is often a sign of difficulty with digesting proteins. Reactions to certain beans and not others are often related to the complexity of the protein compounds in the bean, so you can have reactions to some beans but not to others.

Additional *Information*

A common cause for sensitivity to beans tends to be SIBO, small intestinal bacterial overgrowth, which disrupts the delicate balance of gut flora, creates inflammation, and makes digestion difficult.

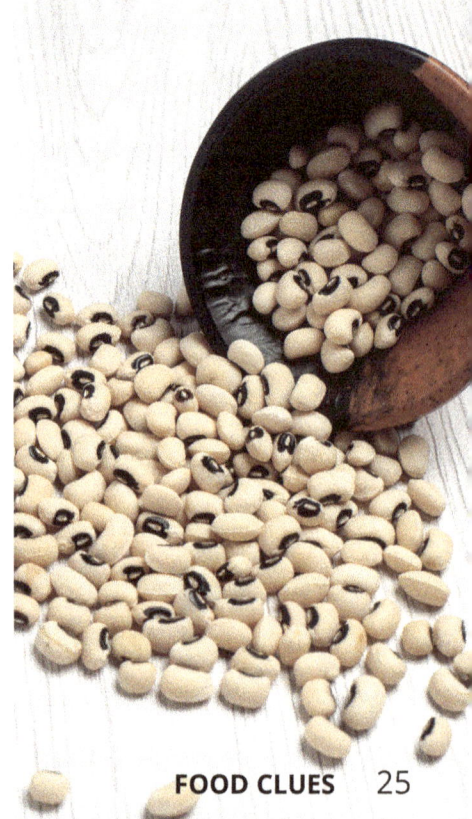

FOOD CLUES

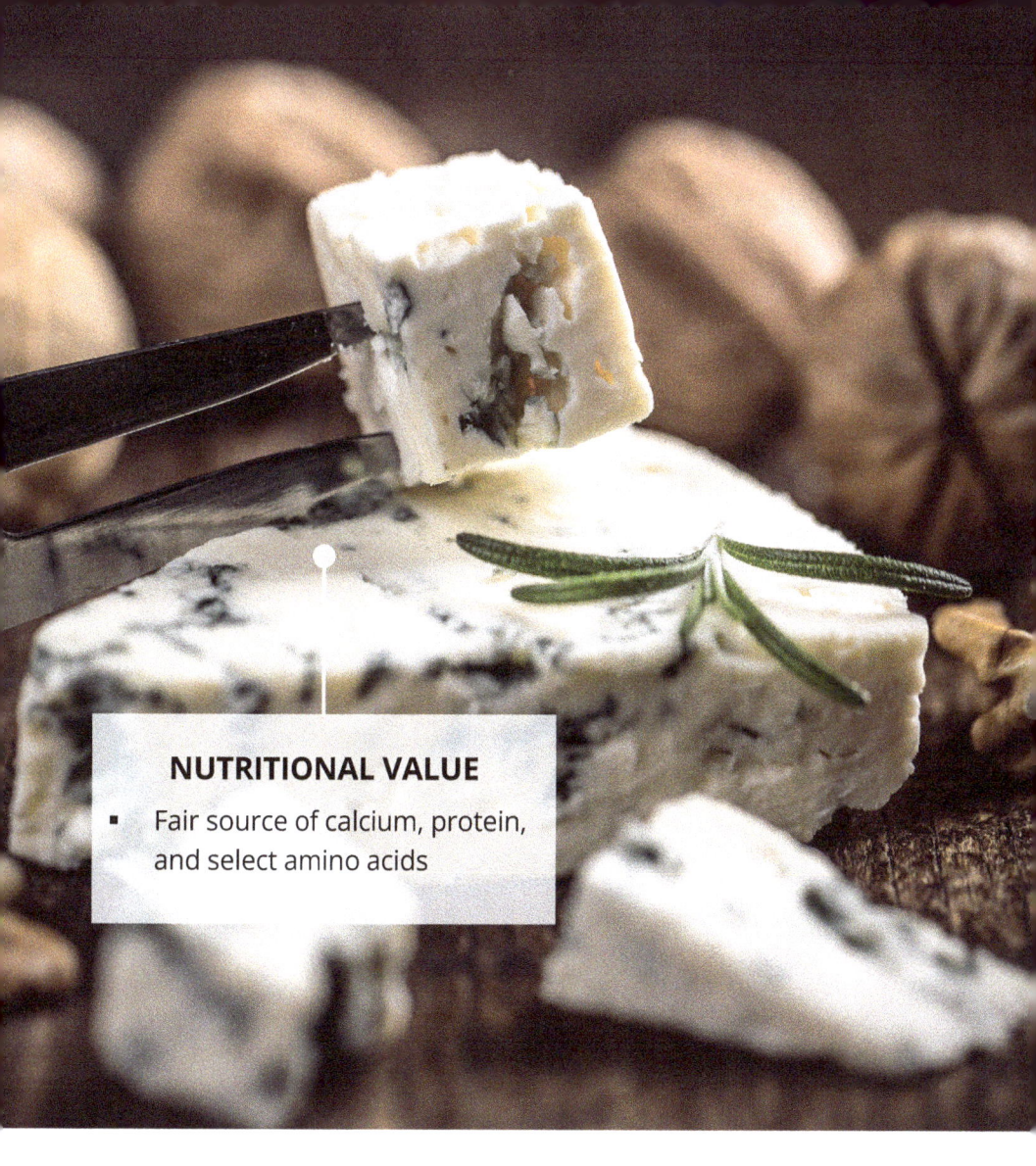

NUTRITIONAL VALUE

- Fair source of calcium, protein, and select amino acids

04 Blue Cheese

Common Avoidance *Responses*

- Headache after smelling
- Nausea after smelling
- Gas
- Bloating
- Abdominal discomfort
- Lip or tongue swelling
- Hives or other skin reactions

Food Clue *Category*

- Elevated germ load
- Unbalanced immune performance

Additional *Information*

As mold is a part of the fungus family, reactions to blue cheese can also be present in those with a fungal overload in their gut flora or a fungal infection.

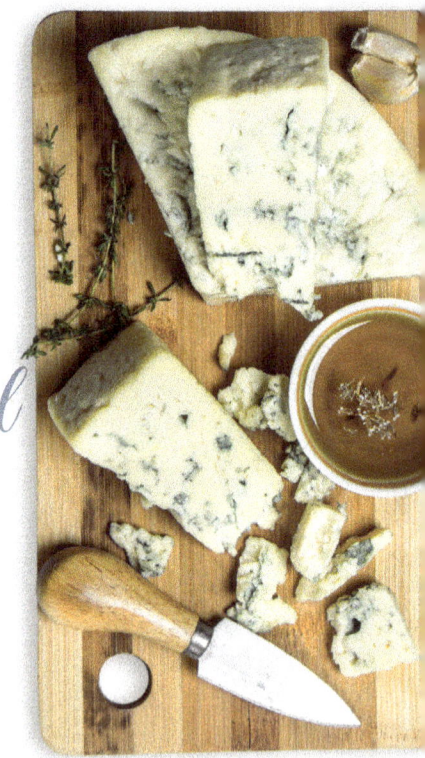

Food Clue *Explained*

Some may react to blue cheese due to its milk properties, meaning they would likely react to other dairy products. But those who react to blue cheese with no history of reacting to dairy products may be doing so due to elevated mold levels in their system. The blue deposits in the cheese are a strain of mold and avoidance of blue cheese can indicate a lingering mold infection in the system.

HEALTH CONCERNS

- Candida overgrowth
- Yeast infection
- Autoimmune conditions

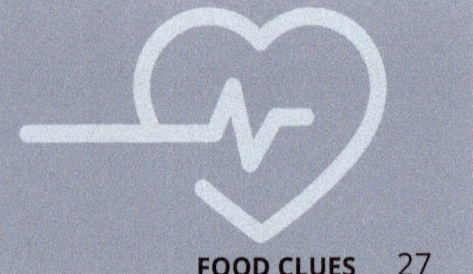

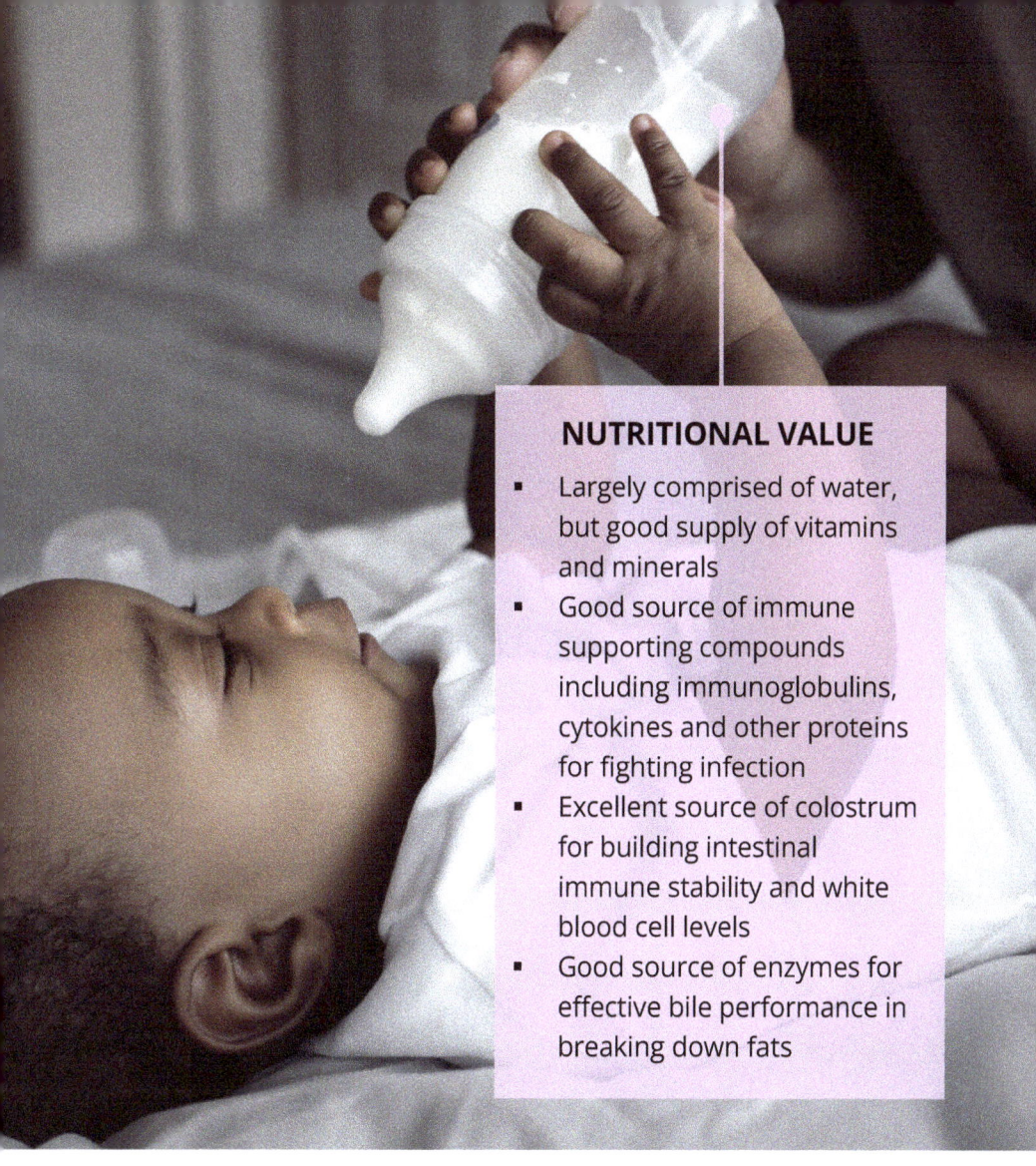

NUTRITIONAL VALUE

- Largely comprised of water, but good supply of vitamins and minerals
- Good source of immune supporting compounds including immunoglobulins, cytokines and other proteins for fighting infection
- Excellent source of colostrum for building intestinal immune stability and white blood cell levels
- Good source of enzymes for effective bile performance in breaking down fats

05 Breast Milk

Common Avoidance *Responses*

- General avoidance or irritability during feeding
- Bloated stomach
- Excessive regurgitation or vomiting
- Colic or croup
- Rash, particularly around the mouth or across the stomach

Food Clue *Category*

- Infection or toxicity

HEALTH CONCERNS

- Beginning of food avoidances and reactions due to poor digestive system integrity and decreased availability of compounds to reduce germs and toxins associated with foods as they are introduced (e.g., egg, dairy, soy allergies).

Food Clue *Explained*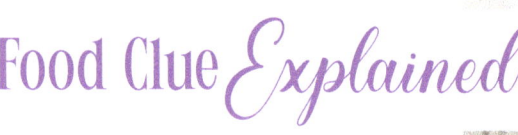

Just as nutrients are passed from mother to child through breast milk, infections and toxic compounds can be transferred as well. If the mother has a significant infectious or toxic load, the baby's natural reaction may be to avoid breast milk as a protective mechanism to prevent further exposure.

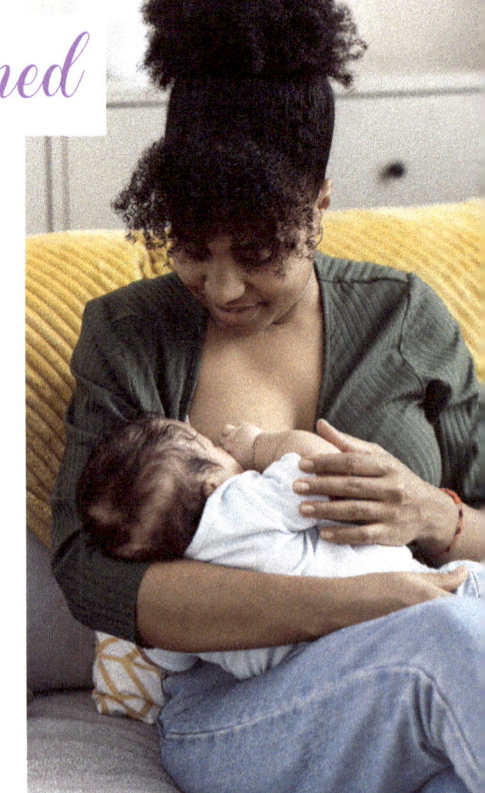

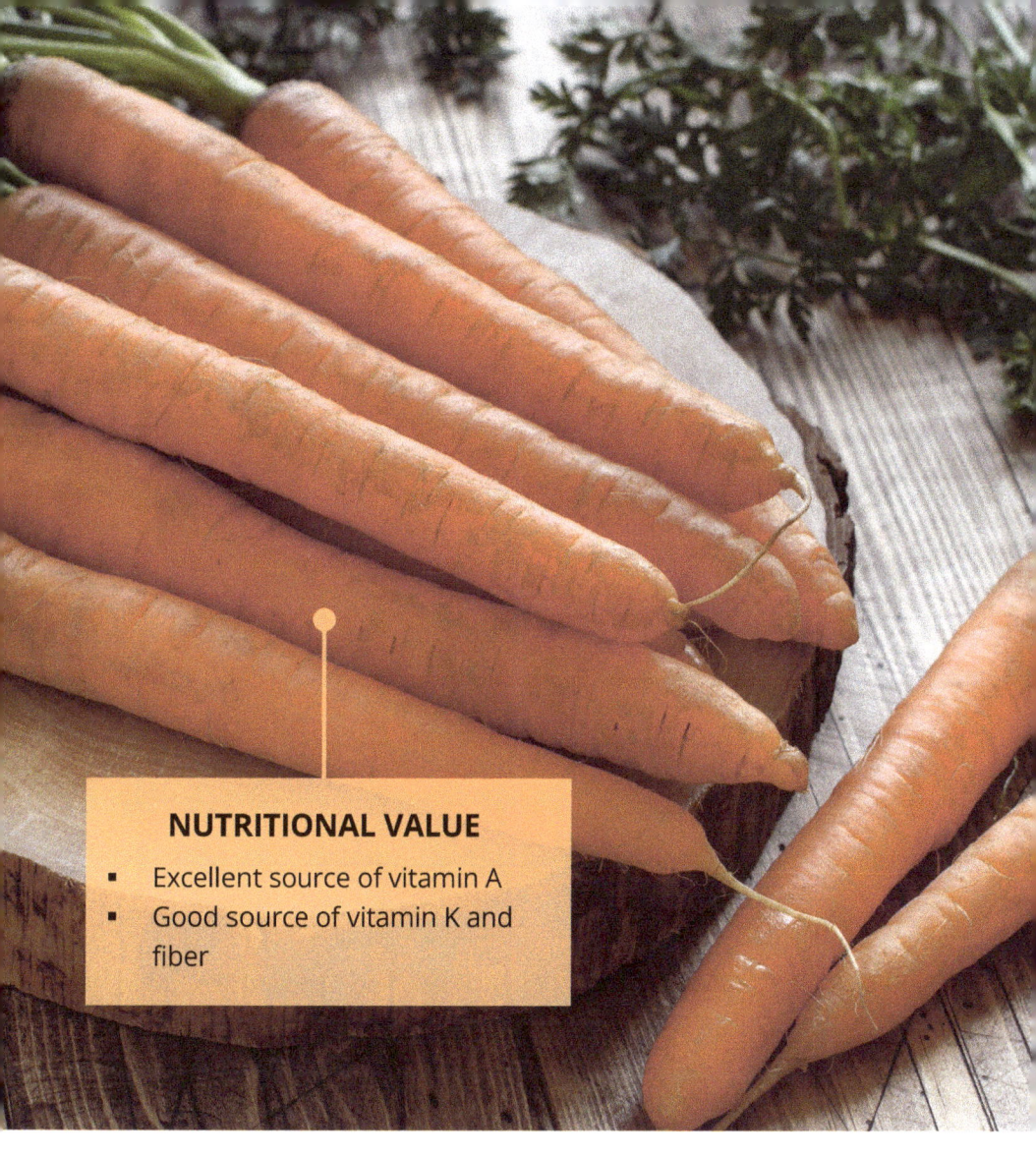

NUTRITIONAL VALUE
- Excellent source of vitamin A
- Good source of vitamin K and fiber

06 Carrots

Common Avoidance *Responses*

- Gas
- Bloating
- Abdominal discomfort

Food Clue *Category*

- Poor nutrient absorption
- Poor protein digestion

HEALTH CONCERNS

- Liver or gallbladder dysfunction
- Difficulty losing weight
- Chronic constipation
- Digestive conditions, including irritable bowel syndrome, Crohn's disease, and celiac disease

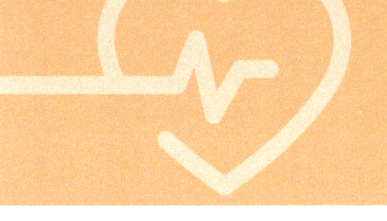

Food Clue *Explained*

There are three typical causes of carrot sensitivity:

1. Poor breakdown of vitamin A in the liver
2. Difficulty with fiber breakdown and absorption
3. Difficulty with protein breakdown, as carrots have specific protein compounds in them associated with sensitivity and allergic reaction (e.g., profilin protein)

Any of these issues within the digestive process can create an avoidance and reaction to carrots when consumed.

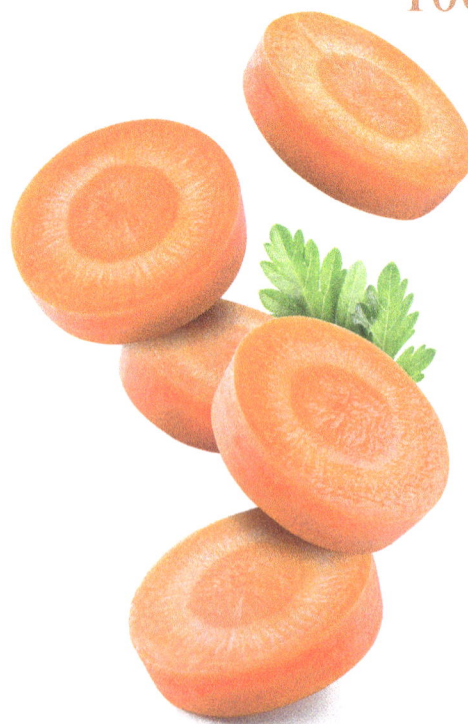

FOOD CLUES 31

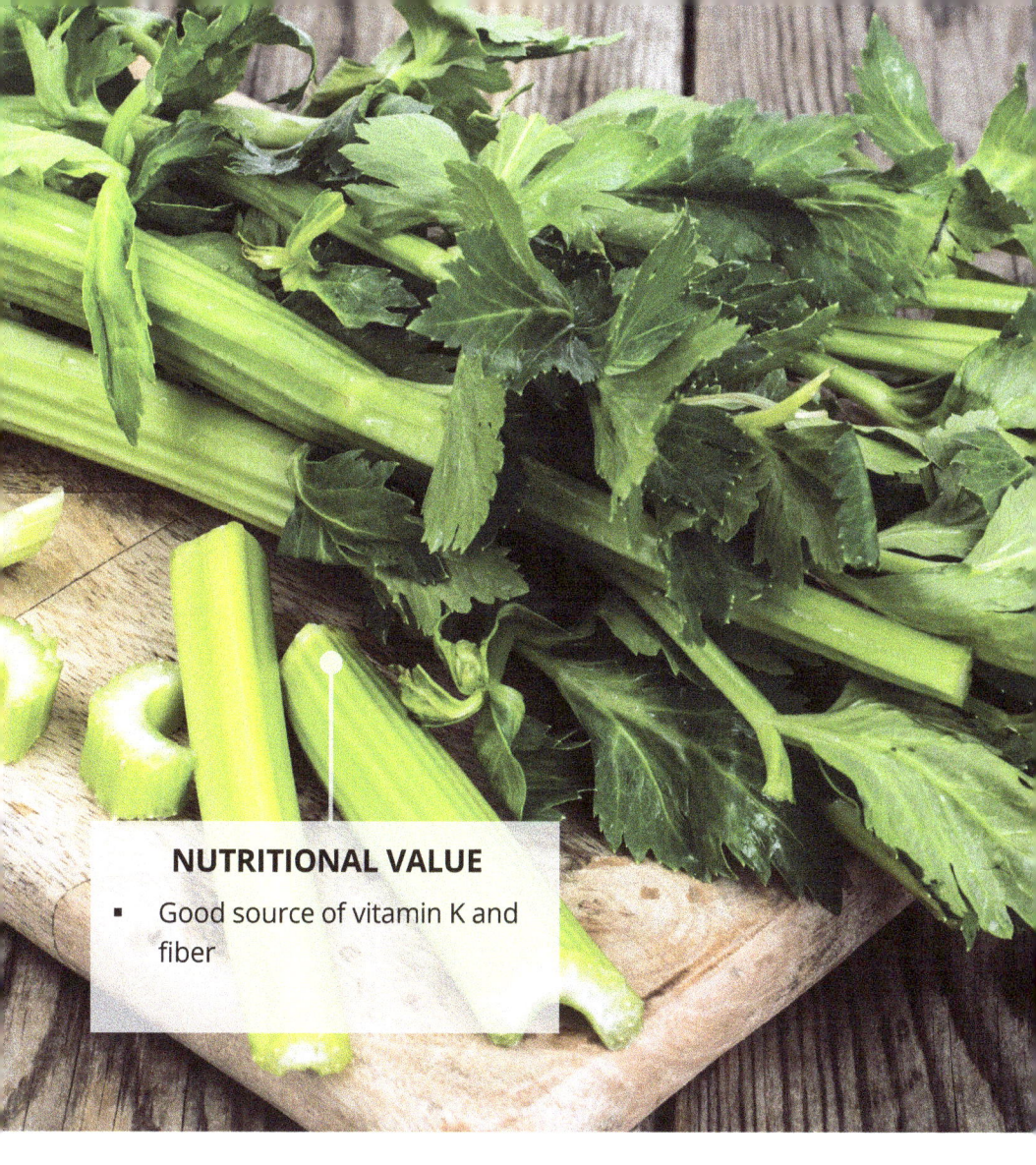

NUTRITIONAL VALUE
- Good source of vitamin K and fiber

07 Celery

Common Avoidance *Responses*

- Gas
- Bloating
- Abdominal discomfort
- Lip or tongue swelling
- Hives or other skin reactions

Food Clue *Category*

- Poor nutrient absorption
- Poor protein digestion

HEALTH CONCERNS

- Liver or gallbladder dysfunction
- Difficulty losing weight
- Chronic constipation
- Digestive conditions, including irritable bowel syndrome, Crohn's disease, and celiac disease

Food Clue *Explained*

There are two typical causes of celery sensitivity:

1. Poor breakdown of vitamin K in the liver
2. Difficulty with protein breakdown, as celery has specific protein compounds in them associated with sensitivity and allergic reaction (e.g., profilin protein)

Any of these issues within the digestive process can create a reaction to celery when consumed.

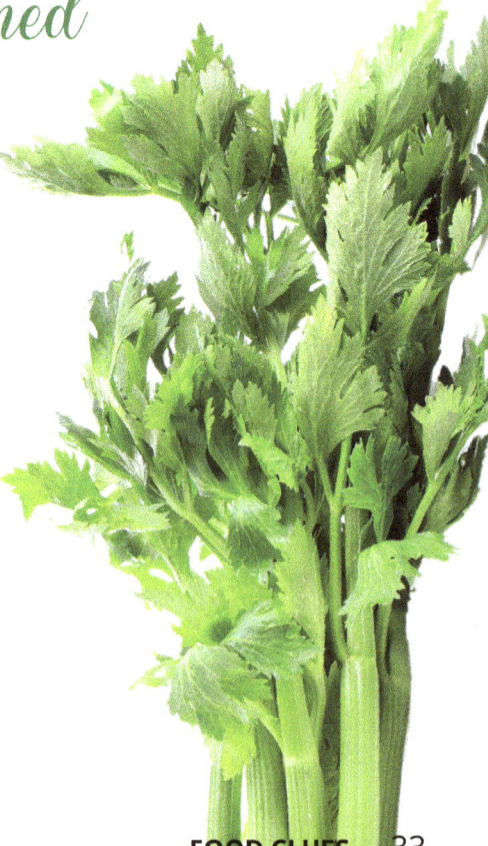

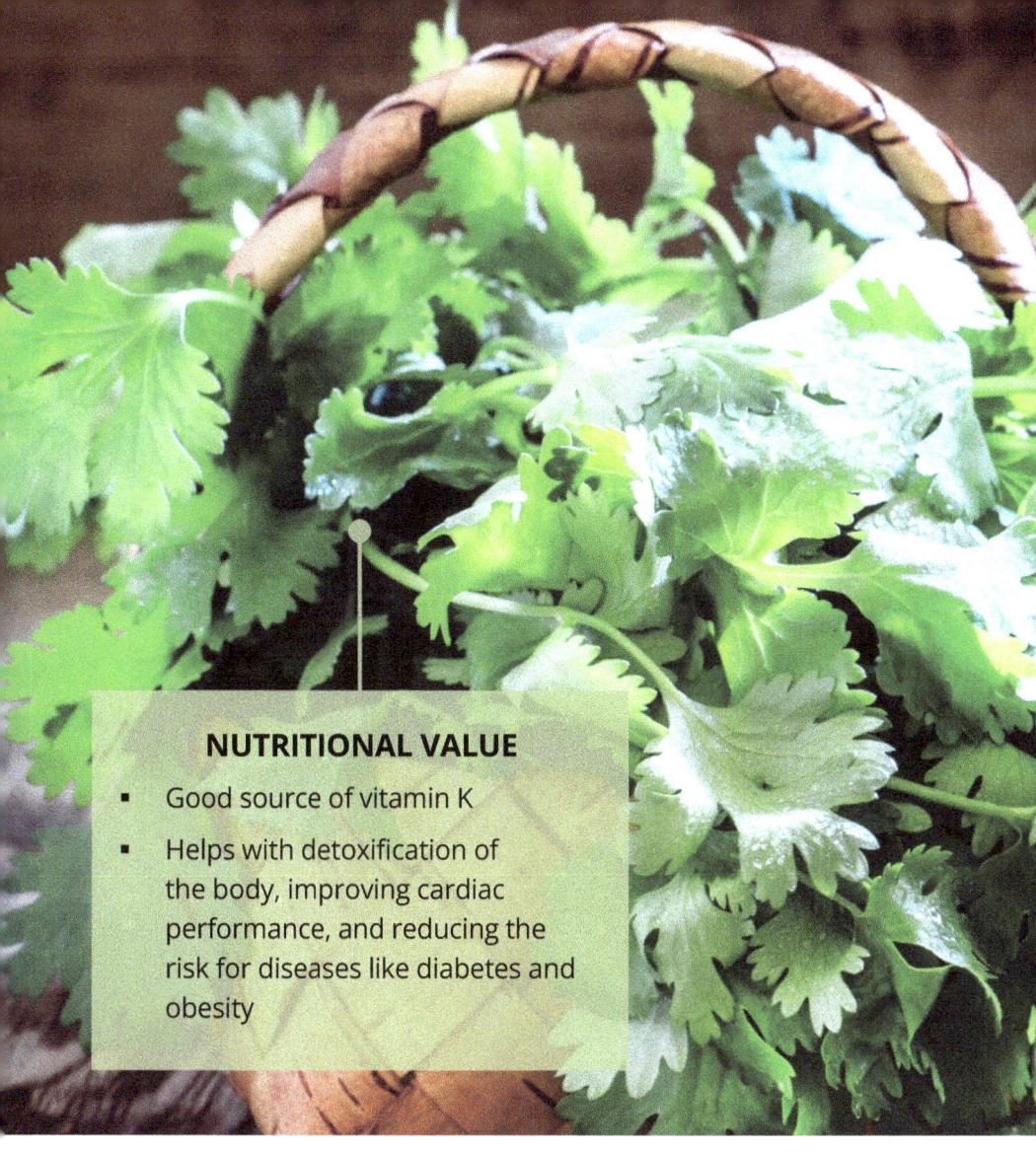

NUTRITIONAL VALUE

- Good source of vitamin K
- Helps with detoxification of the body, improving cardiac performance, and reducing the risk for diseases like diabetes and obesity

08 Cilantro

Common Avoidance *Responses*

- General avoidance (People will say it tastes like soap)

Food Clue *Category*

- Poor nutrient absorption
- Poor general digestion

Additional *Information*

Infection or toxicity, particularly affecting the digestive tract, is often a major culprit of cilantro avoidance.

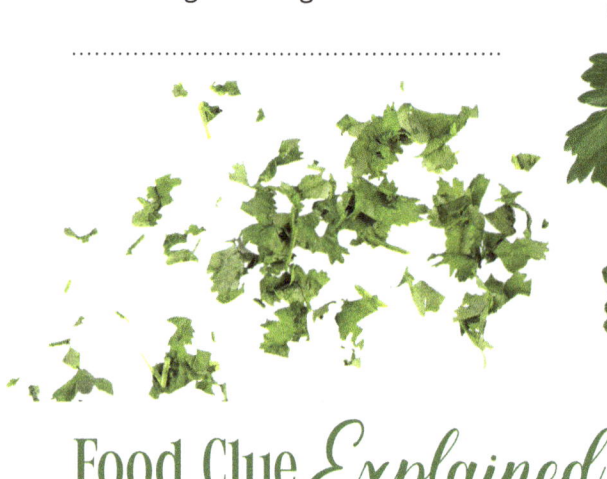

Food Clue *Explained*

Cilantro is high in profilins, which are a type of plant protein. Avoidance of cilantro can be a sign of difficulty with protein digestion and managing acids which are the building blocks of proteins.

Cilantro also has properties that aid with detoxification, especially of metals. Avoidance of cilantro can indicate difficulty with the detoxification process, which largely occurs in the liver.

HEALTH CONCERNS

- Liver or gallbladder dysfunction
- Thyroid dysfunction
- Autoimmune conditions

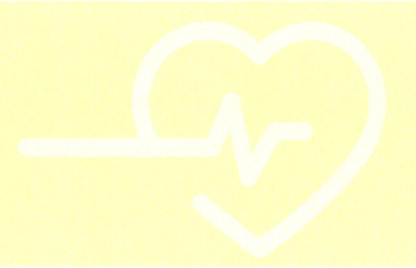

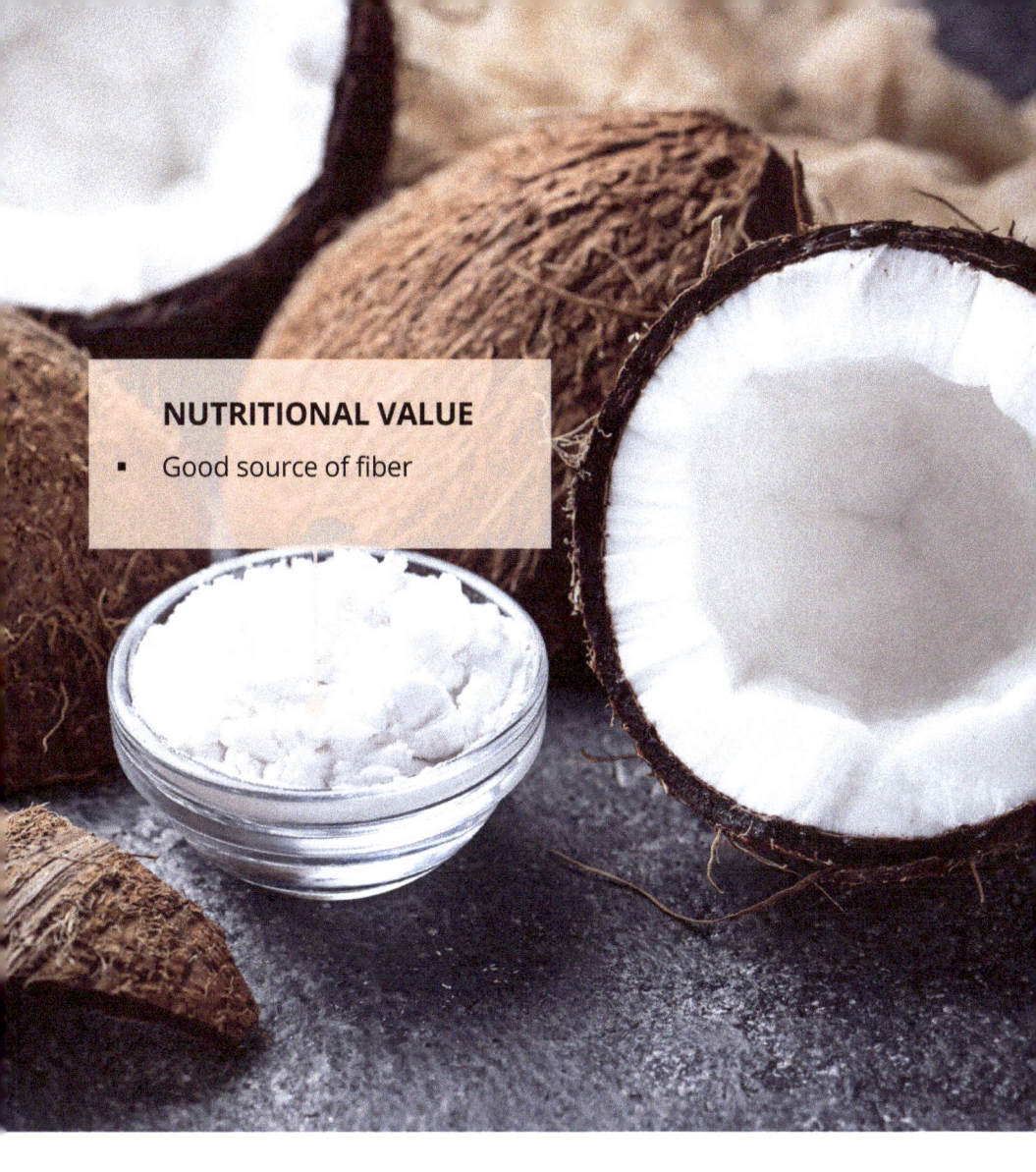

NUTRITIONAL VALUE
- Good source of fiber

09 Coconut

Common Avoidance *Responses*

- Gas
- Bloating
- Abdominal discomfort

Food Clue *Category*

- Unbalanced gut bacteria levels
- Elevated germ load

HEALTH CONCERNS

- Menstrual cycle dysfunction or conditions including heavy bleeding, missed cycles, endometriosis, and polycystic ovary syndrome (PCOS)
- Chronic constipation
- Digestive conditions including irritable bowel syndrome, Crohn's disease, and celiac disease

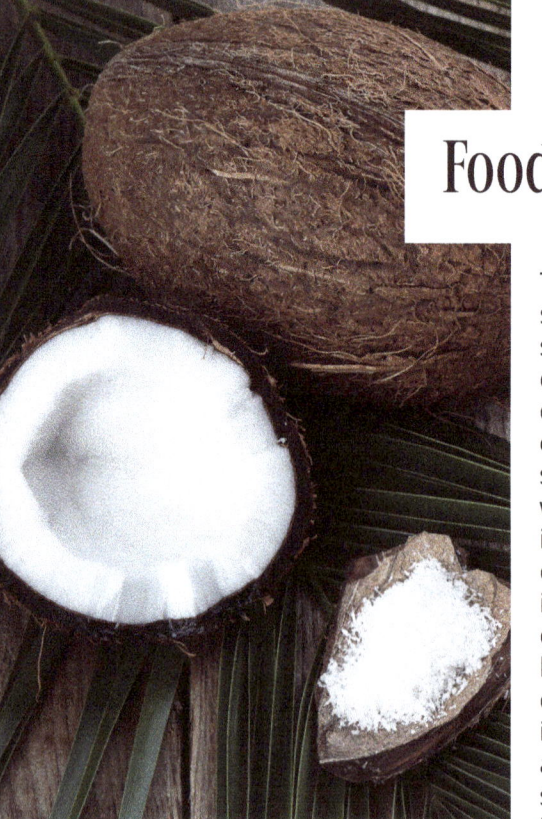

Food Clue *Explained*

The most common cause of coconut sensitivity is its high amount of saturated fats. One daily serving of coconut is estimated to have 125% of the daily value requirement of saturated fat. Diets high in saturated fats have been associated with bacterial infection, gut flora imbalance (also called dysbiosis), and even hormone and neurotransmitter imbalances, including imbalanced estrogen, serotonin, and dopamine levels. Avoidance or reactions to coconut may be a sign that the body is overloaded with too much bacteria and is restricting acceptance of substances that would contribute to its growth.

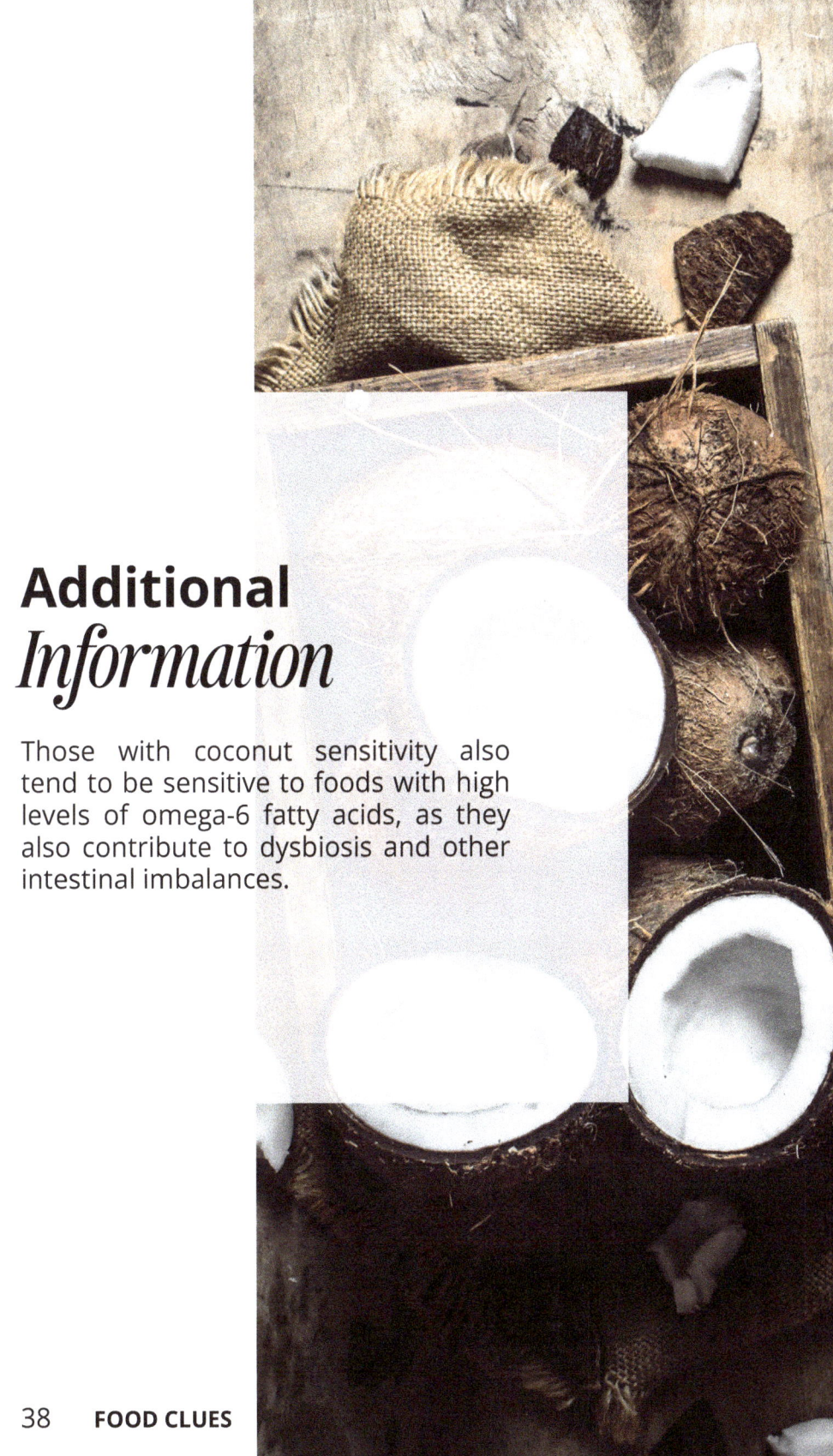

Additional
Information

Those with coconut sensitivity also tend to be sensitive to foods with high levels of omega-6 fatty acids, as they also contribute to dysbiosis and other intestinal imbalances.

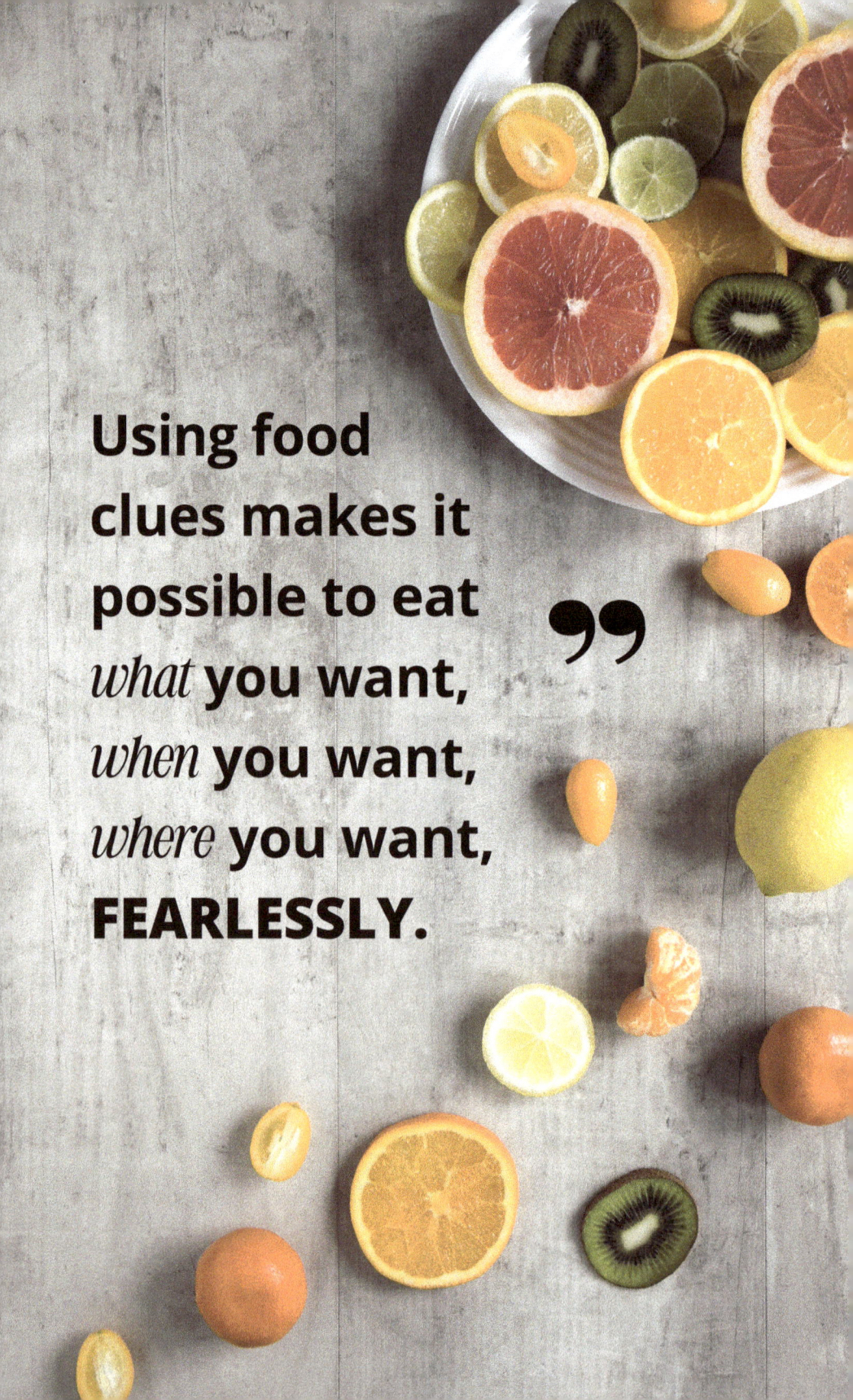

> **Using food clues makes it possible to eat** *what* **you want,** *when* **you want,** *where* **you want, FEARLESSLY.**

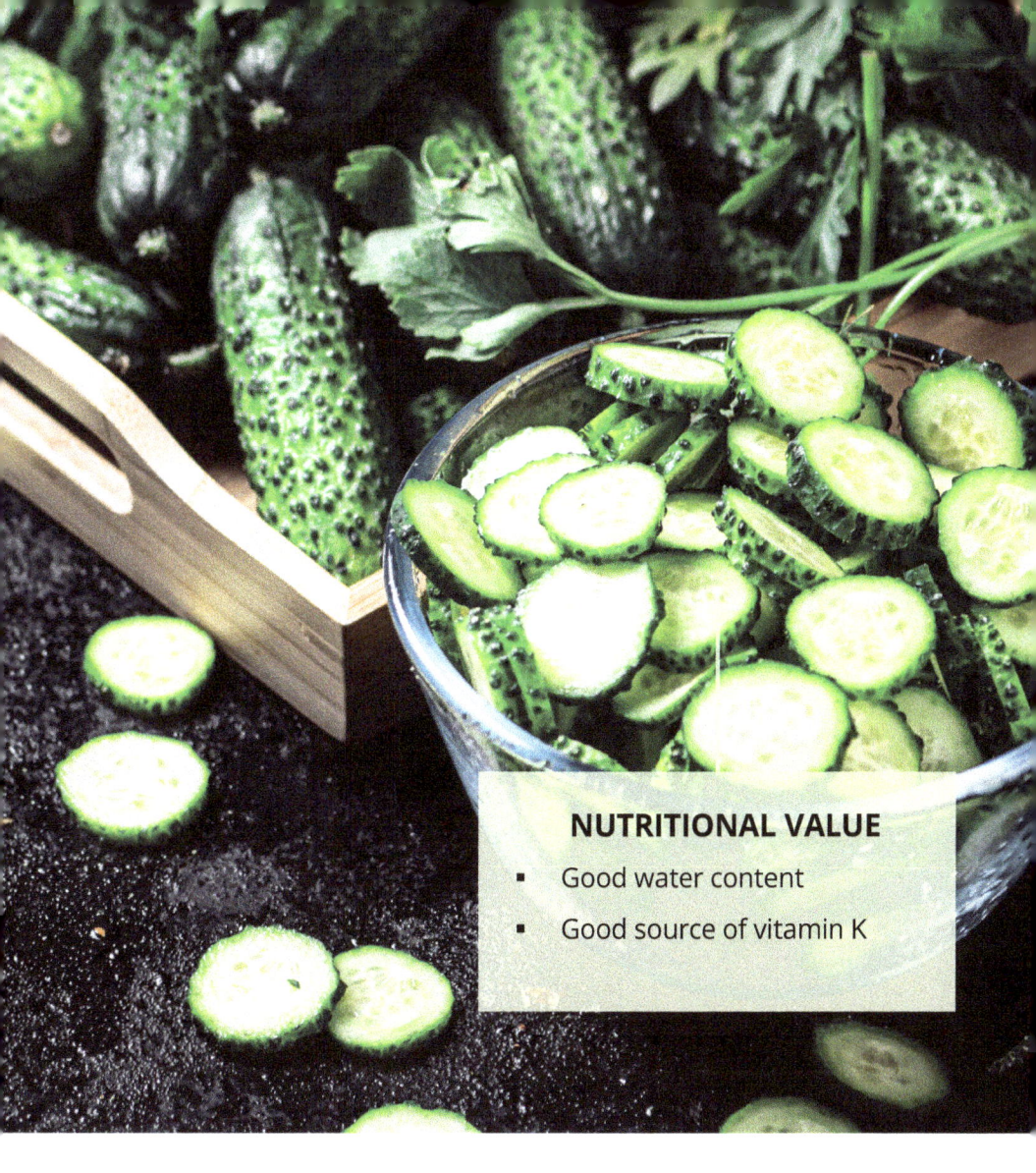

NUTRITIONAL VALUE

- Good water content
- Good source of vitamin K

10 Cucumbers

Common Avoidance *Responses*

- General avoidance

Food Clue *Category*

- Poor protein digestion

Food Clue *Explained*

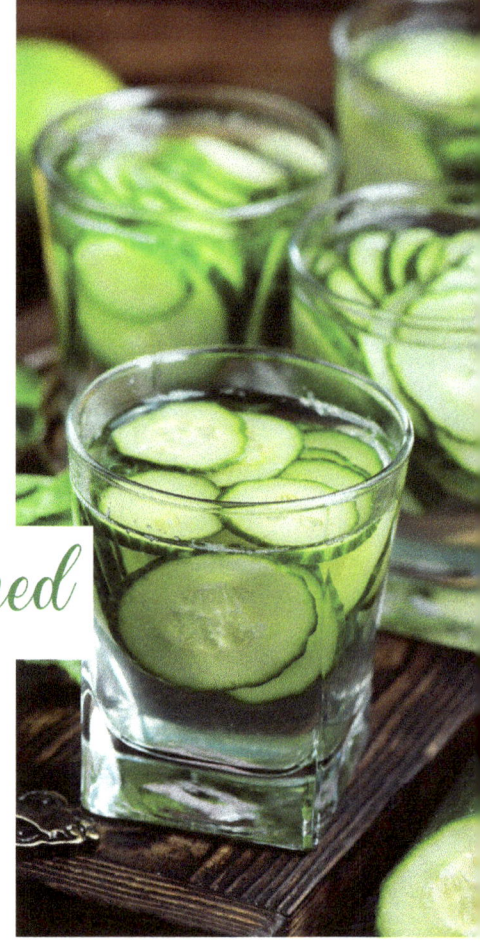

Cucumbers are high in lectins and profilins, which are both proteins. So avoidance of cucumbers can be a sign of difficulty with protein digestion and managing acids.

It's been suggested that avoidance of cucumber is also associated with dysfunction of the TAS2R38 gene, which controls the detection of bitterness and potentially poisonous compounds. This detection triggers the release of digestive juices to aid in breaking down food or eliminating harmful compounds from the body. When gene performance is low, the "bitter trigger" isn't activated and digestion can become problematic.

Additional *Information*

Infection or toxicity, particularly affecting the digestive tract, is often a major culprit of cucumber avoidance.

HEALTH CONCERNS

- Digestive conditions including irritable bowel syndrome, Crohn's disease, celiac disease
- Emotional and mental health imbalances including anxiety, depression, autism, attention deficit disorder, attention deficit hyperactivity disorder

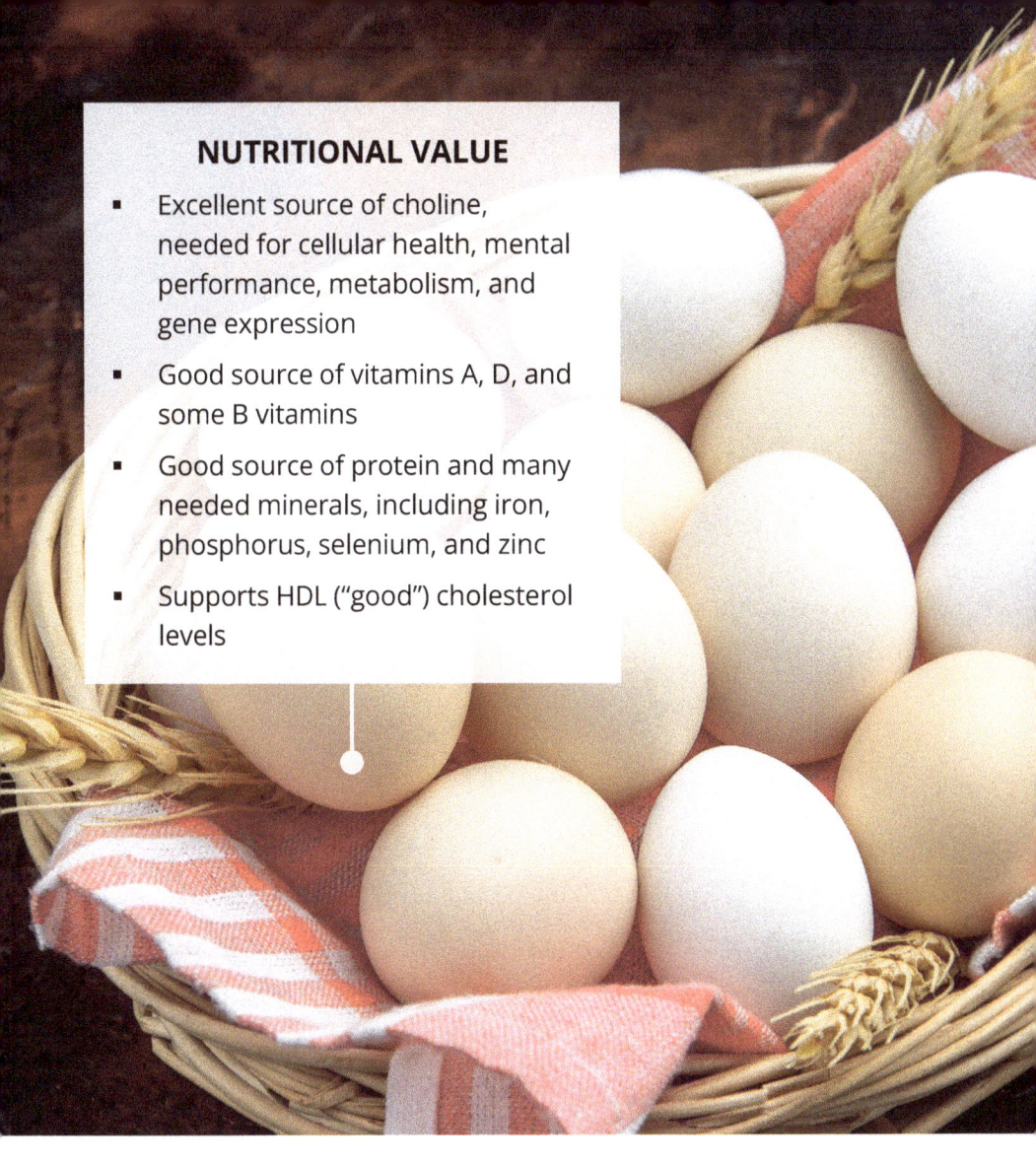

NUTRITIONAL VALUE

- Excellent source of choline, needed for cellular health, mental performance, metabolism, and gene expression
- Good source of vitamins A, D, and some B vitamins
- Good source of protein and many needed minerals, including iron, phosphorus, selenium, and zinc
- Supports HDL ("good") cholesterol levels

11 Eggs

Common Avoidance *Responses*

- Gas
- Bloating
- Abdominal discomfort
- Nausea

Food Clue *Category*

- Poor protein digestion
- Poor liver function

HEALTH CONCERNS

- Liver or gallbladder dysfunction
- Thyroid dysfunction
- Small intestinal bacterial overgrowth (SIBO)
- Digestive conditions including irritable bowel syndrome, Crohn's disease, celiac disease

Food Clue *Explained*

Reactions to egg whites suggest more difficulty with protein digestion, while reactions to the yolk suggest poor liver function, particularly for managing sulfur levels and transporting it where needed for body processes. Reactions can also suggest difficulty with methylation, a key process that transfers hydrogen and carbon compounds throughout the body, influencing nearly every chemical reaction that takes place in each of our organs and body systems.

Allergy *Stats*

- Eggs are considered a top allergy by the National Institute of Health
- About 2% of children have an egg allergy, typically outgrown by adulthood

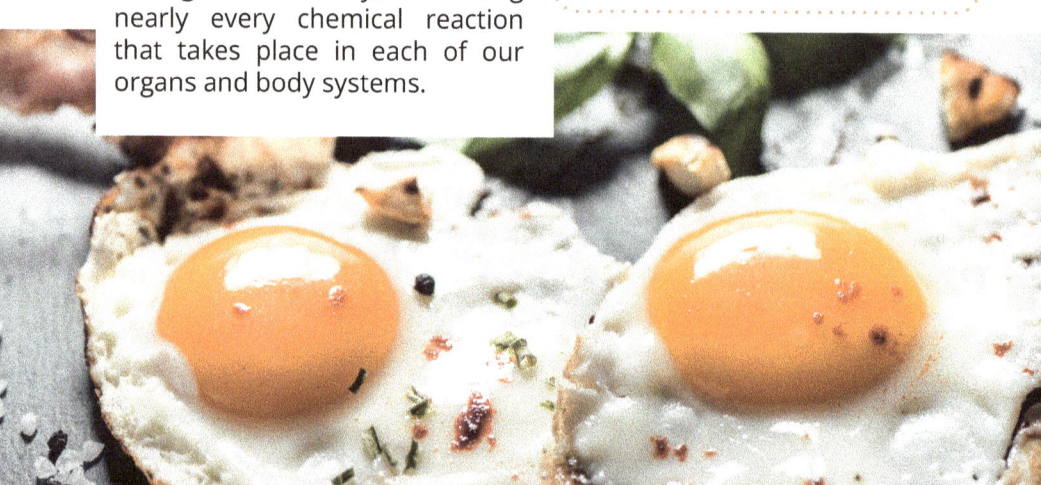

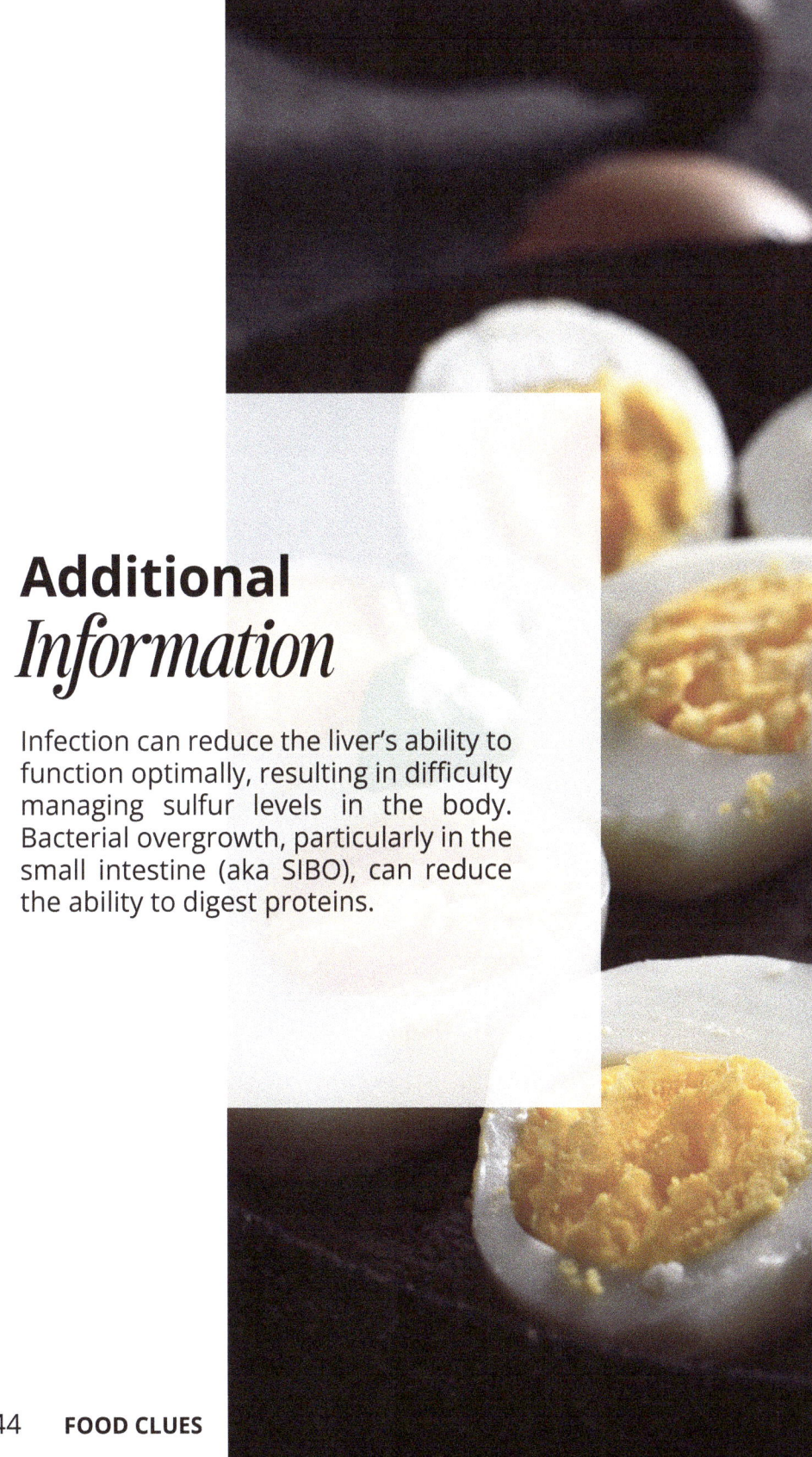

Additional
Information

Infection can reduce the liver's ability to function optimally, resulting in difficulty managing sulfur levels in the body. Bacterial overgrowth, particularly in the small intestine (aka SIBO), can reduce the ability to digest proteins.

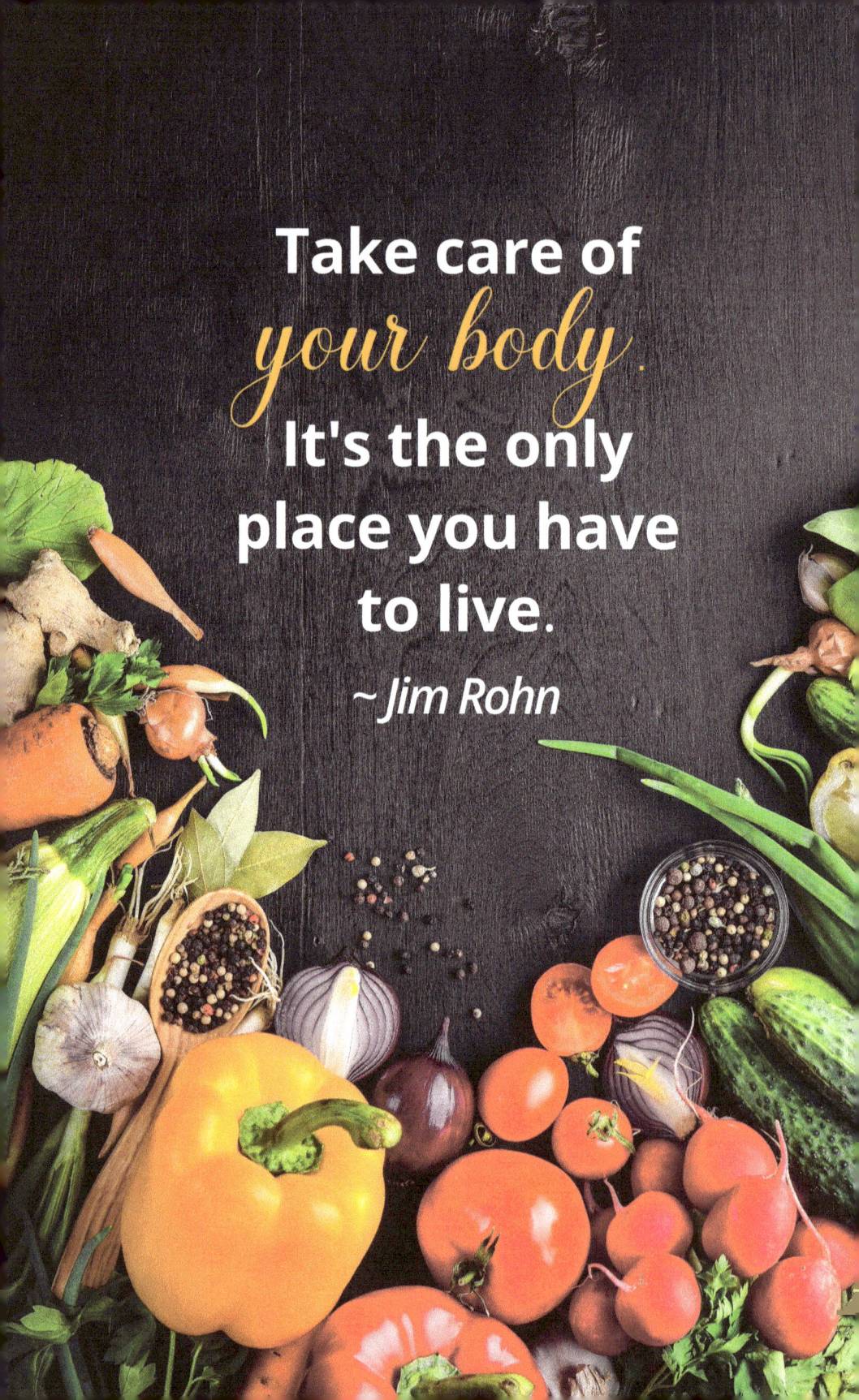

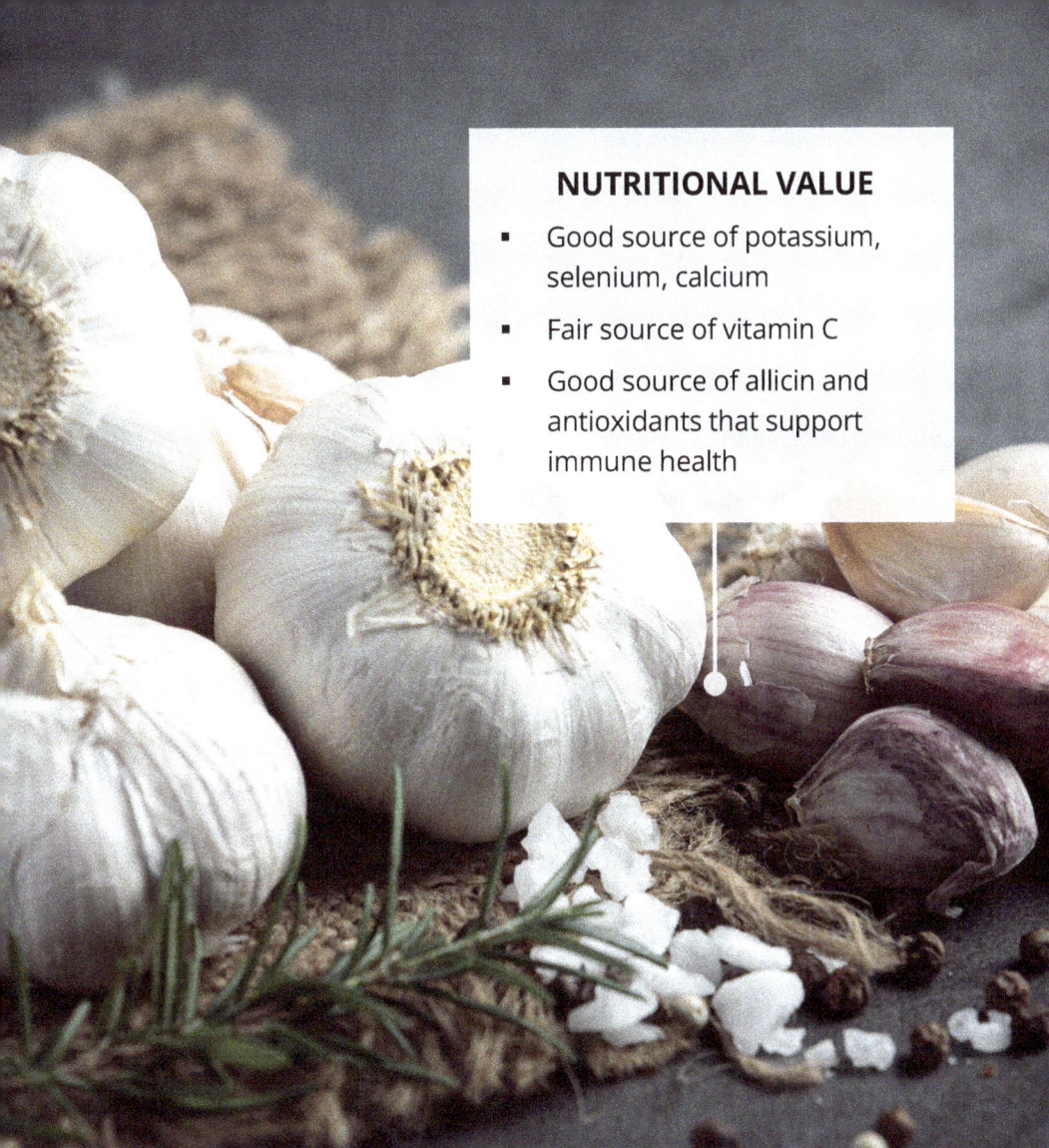

NUTRITIONAL VALUE

- Good source of potassium, selenium, calcium
- Fair source of vitamin C
- Good source of allicin and antioxidants that support immune health

12 Garlic

Common Avoidance *Responses*

- Gas
- Bloating
- Abdominal discomfort

Food Clue *Category*

- Unbalanced immune performance

HEALTH CONCERNS

- Chronic allergy or flu symptoms
- Autoimmune conditions
- Mast cell activation syndrome
- Liver or gallbladder dysfunction

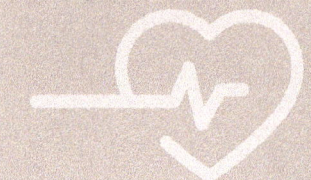

Food Clue *Explained*

A common cause of garlic reactions is elevated histamine levels in the body. Histamines are secondary aids to stimulating stomach acid secretion, reducing inflammation, dilating blood vessels, supporting muscle contractions in the intestines and lungs, and influencing heart rate. If any of the other organs or systems driving those functions become impaired, histamine levels may be boosted as compensation to keep those functions going, and foods high in histamine may be avoided to reduce histamine overload.

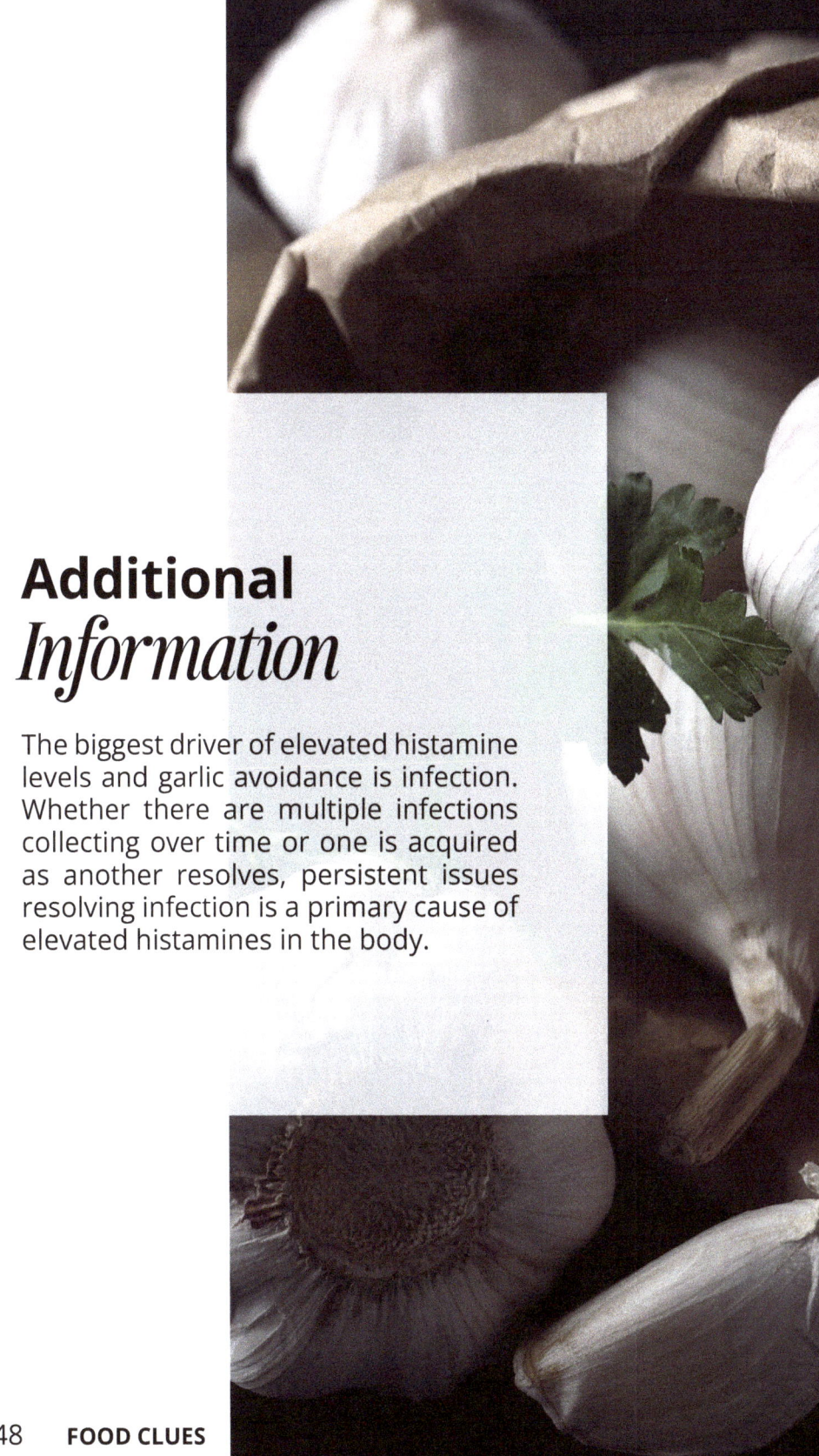

Additional
Information

The biggest driver of elevated histamine levels and garlic avoidance is infection. Whether there are multiple infections collecting over time or one is acquired as another resolves, persistent issues resolving infection is a primary cause of elevated histamines in the body.

> **HEALTH BEGINS WITH UNDERSTANDING YOUR BODY'S FOOD LANGUAGE.**

·········

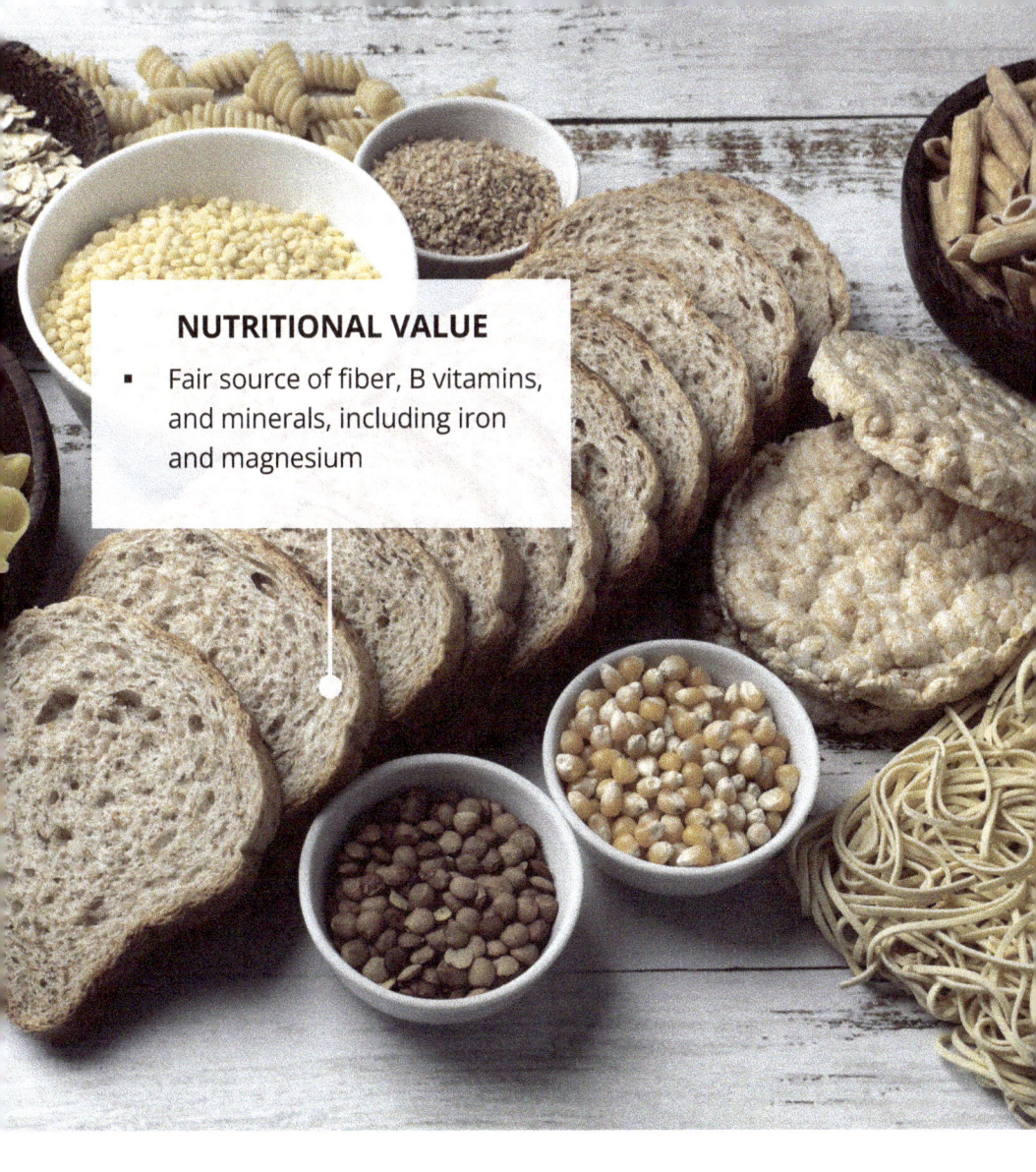

NUTRITIONAL VALUE

- Fair source of fiber, B vitamins, and minerals, including iron and magnesium

13 Gluten

FOOD CLUES

Common Avoidance *Responses*

- Abdominal discomfort
- Gas
- Bloating

Allergy *Stats*

- Wheat is considered a top allergen by the National Institute of Health
- Studies have shown a prevalence of wheat allergy in children of around 0.4 percent, with most showing less reactivity by age twelve.
- Non-celiac gluten sensitivity affects about 6% of the US population.
- Some medical institutes estimate up to eighteen million people in the United States have gluten sensitivity.

Food Clue *Category*

- Poor protein digestion

HEALTH CONCERNS
- Small intestinal bacterial overgrowth (SIBO)

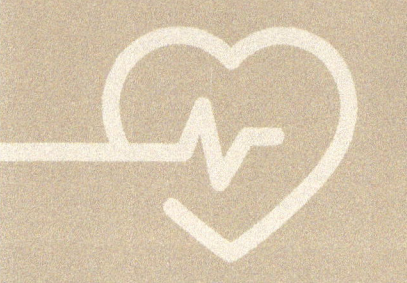
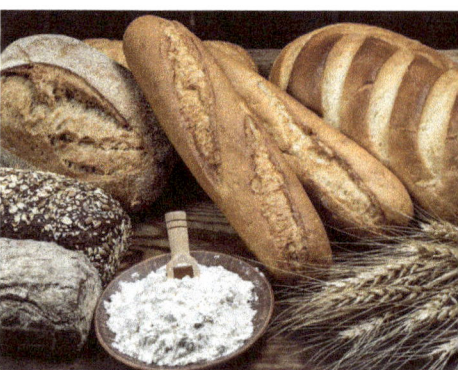

Food Clue *Explained*

Since gluten is a natural protein commonly found in wheat and other grains, reactions to wheat often suggest difficulty with protein digestion. Gluten reactions can also suggest difficulty with acid breakdown or elimination, or indicate an overload of acid, resulting in an avoidance reaction against eating gluten, since the building blocks of proteins are amino acids.

Profilin protein is another common protein found in many plants that pose a challenge in terms of digestion and absorption.

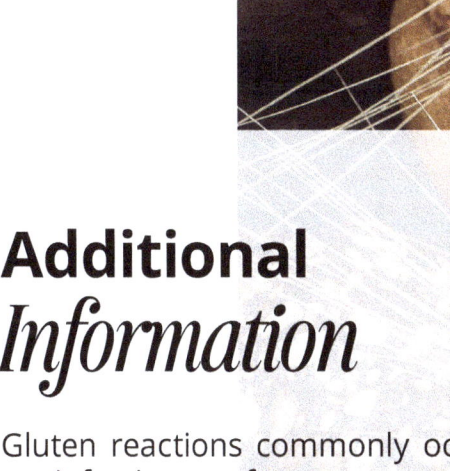

Additional
Information

Gluten reactions commonly occur due to infections, often concentrated in the stomach and small intestine, which disrupt digestion. Gluten reactions could also indicate exposure to acidic chemicals, raising the overall acidity of the body, resulting in avoidance of or reactions to anything acidic.

Allergies to wheat and other foods naturally containing gluten may specifically be in response to the agricultural chemicals used during the growing and preservation processes (e.g., glyphosate).

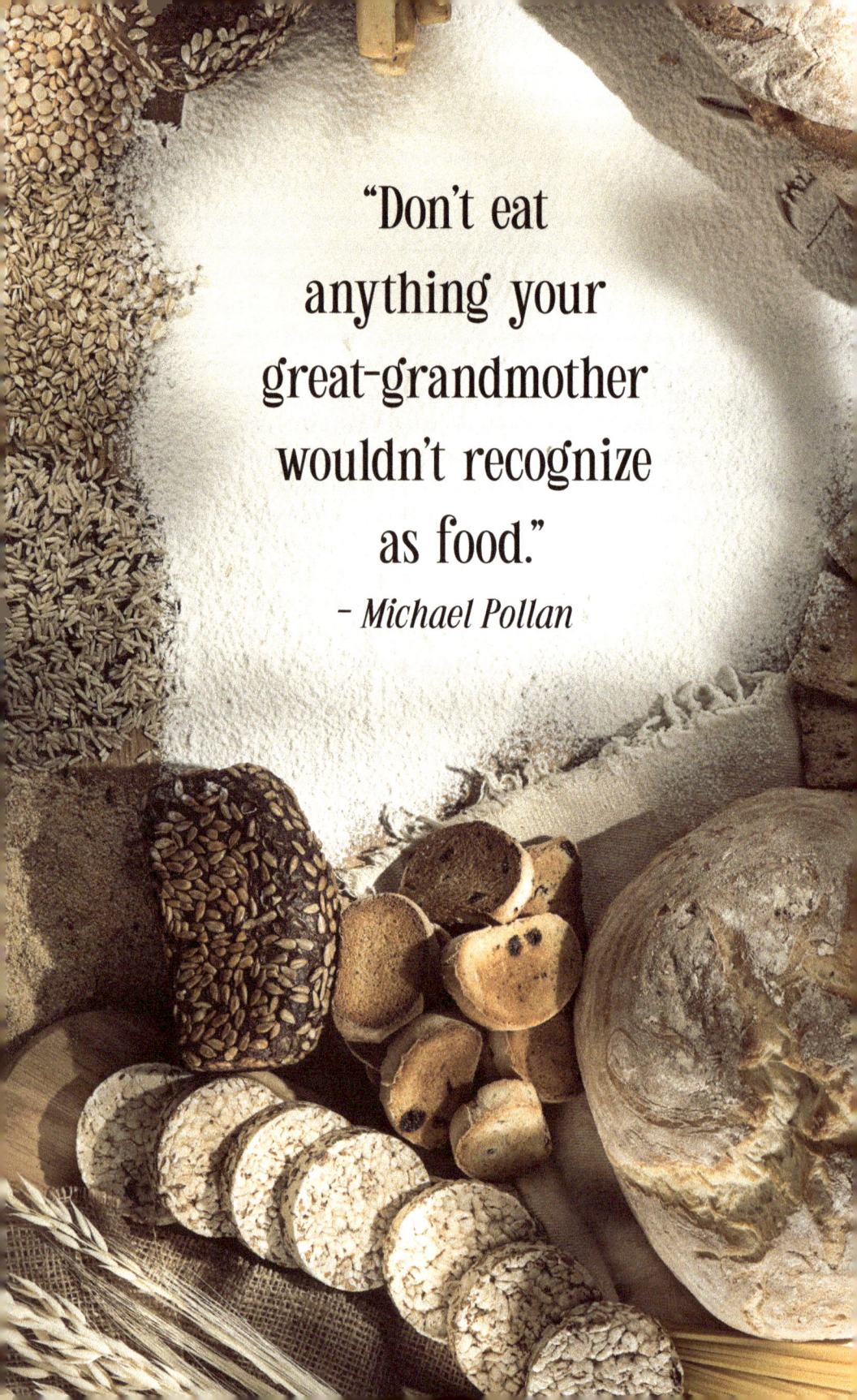

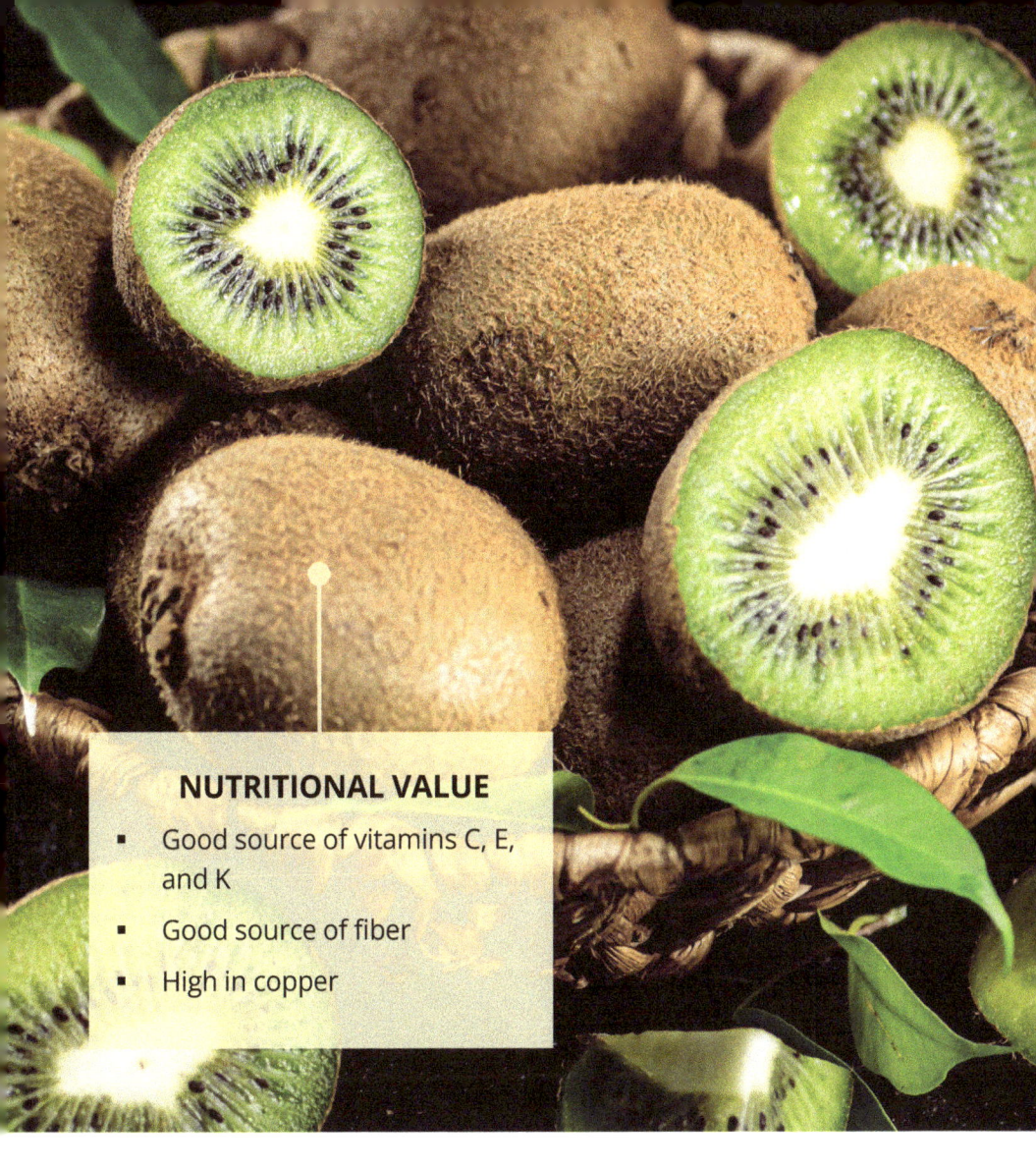

NUTRITIONAL VALUE

- Good source of vitamins C, E, and K
- Good source of fiber
- High in copper

14 Kiwi

Common Avoidance *Responses*

- Lip or tongue swelling
- Itchy skin
- Hives or other skin reactions
- Gas
- Bloating
- Nausea

Food Clue *Category*

- Poor nutrient absorption
- Poor protein digestion
- Metal toxicity

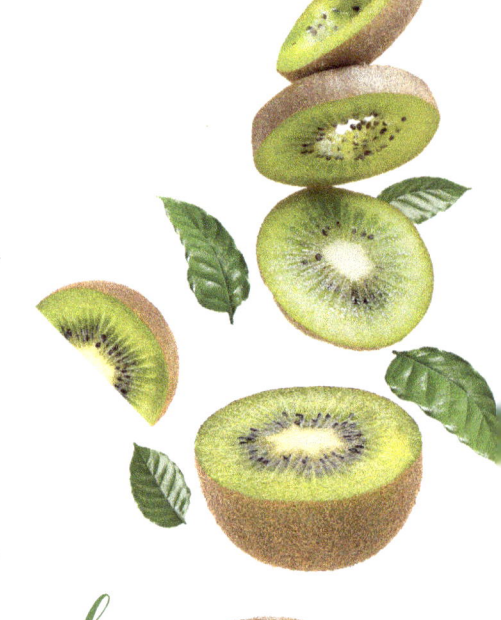

Food Clue *Explained*

Sensitivity and allergic reactions to kiwi can be related to a number of its properties, including the following:

1. Difficulty breaking down plant-specific proteins (e.g., lipid transfer protein, profilin)
2. Difficulty breaking down latex proteins
3. Elevated metal loads in the body

HEALTH CONCERNS

- Liver or gallbladder dysfunction
- Digestive conditions including irritable bowel syndrome, Crohn's disease, celiac disease

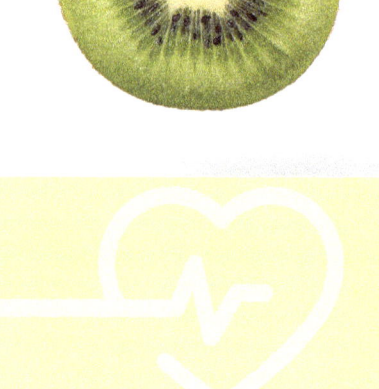

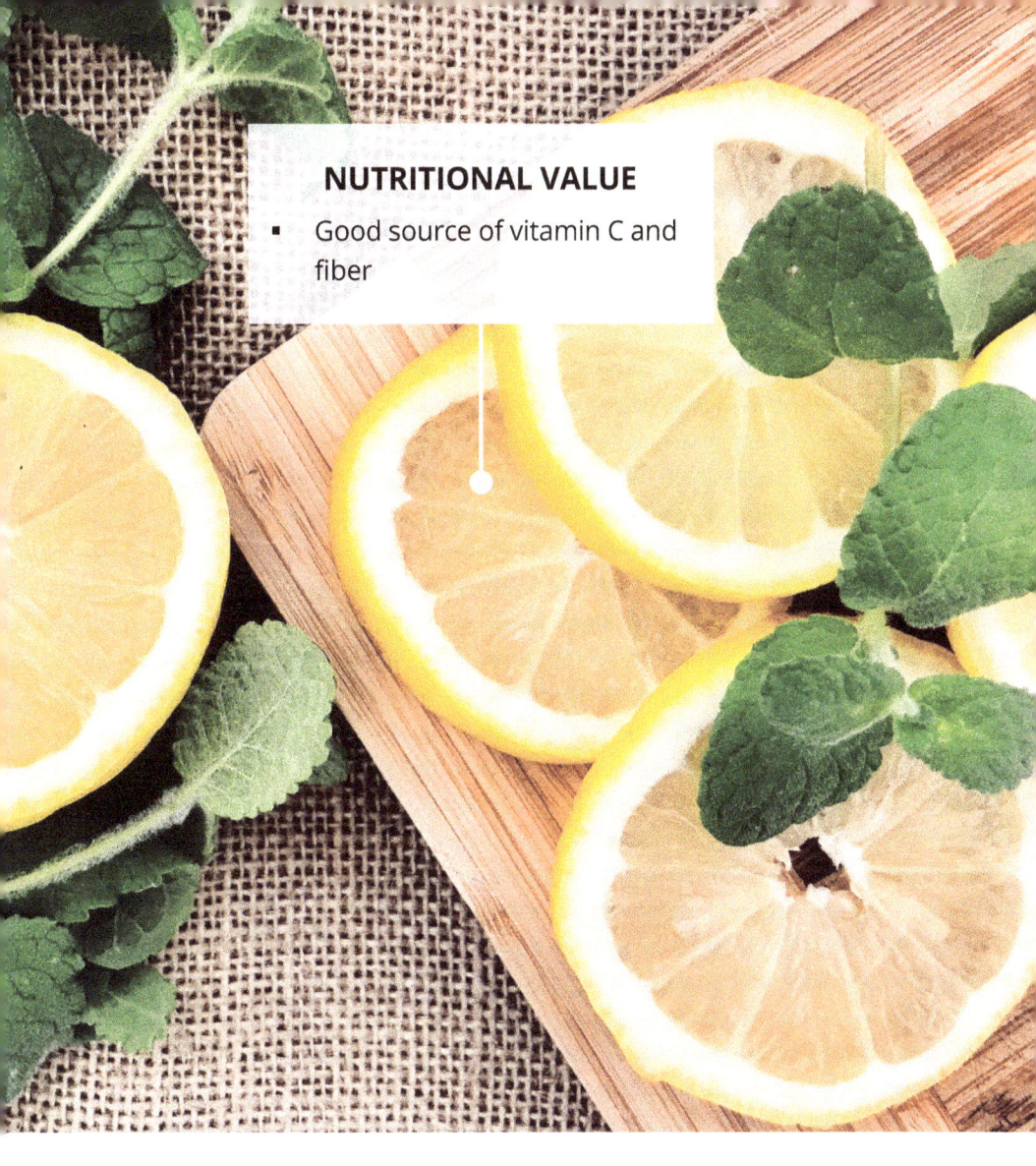

NUTRITIONAL VALUE
- Good source of vitamin C and fiber

15 Lemon

Common Avoidance *Responses*

- General avoidance

Food Clue *Category*

- Poor general digestion
- Poor liver function
- Poor acid management

HEALTH CONCERNS
- Liver or gallbladder dysfunction
- Gastrointestinal ulcers
- Gastroesophageal reflux disease (GERD)

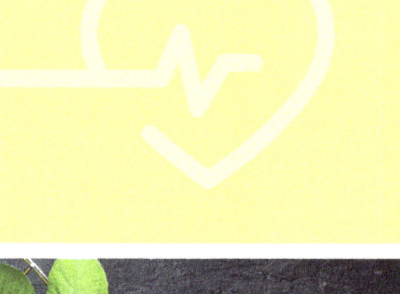

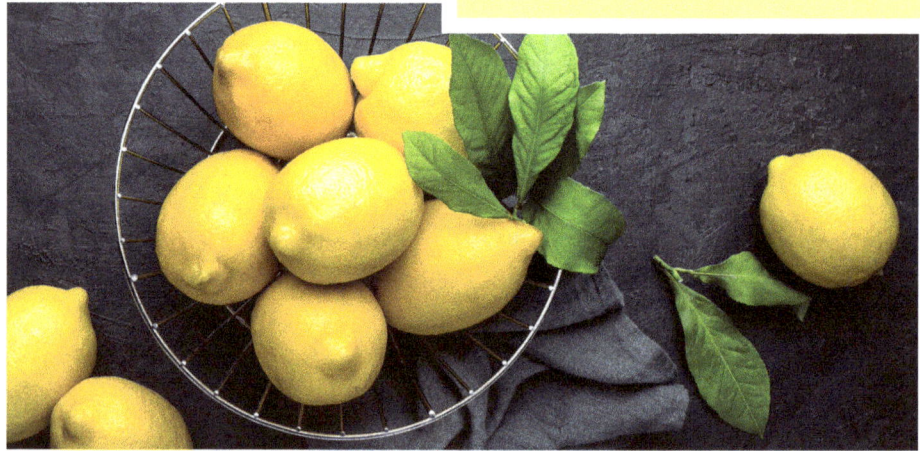

Food Clue *Explained*

Similar to those who avoid tomatoes, many people avoid lemons due to their acidic content. The pH of a lemon averages 2.5, so people who avoid lemon may do so due to thin or inflamed stomach or intestinal lining, which becomes more irritated when acids come into contact with it. An impaired stomach lining may also cause decreased release of bile and other digestive juices, which are typically acidic in nature, resulting in difficulty with the digestion of fats and other substances.

Additional
Information

Although traditional allergies are rare, they are often linked to profilin, a common plant protein known to create difficulty with digestion, resulting in sensitivity and avoidance.

Lemons and other citrus fruits also contain limonene, a compound found in the peel of the fruit, known to irritate skin as its primary avoidance response. Limonene is an antioxidant which supports liver performance in the detoxification of waste, so avoidance via skin reaction could indicate poor liver function.

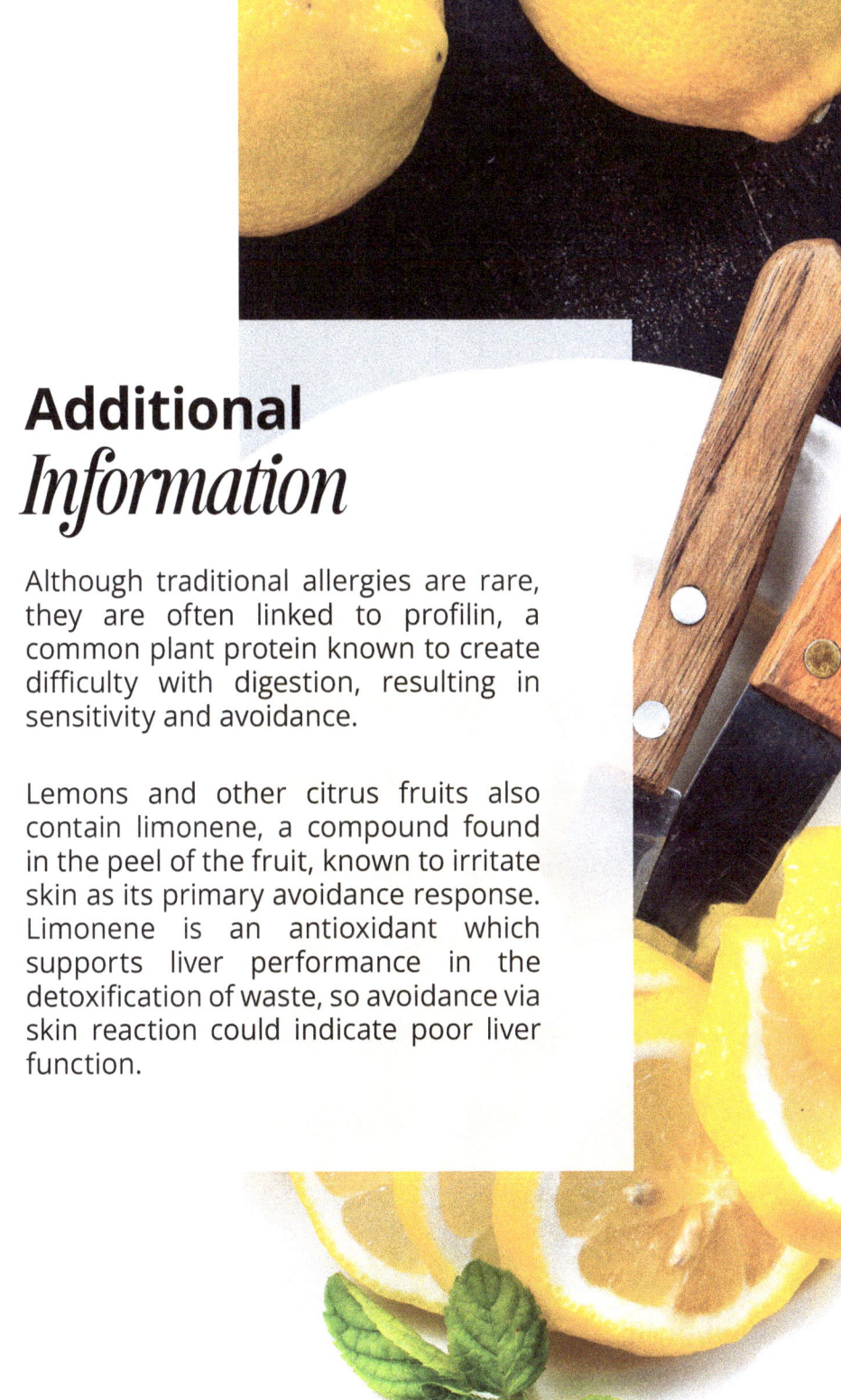

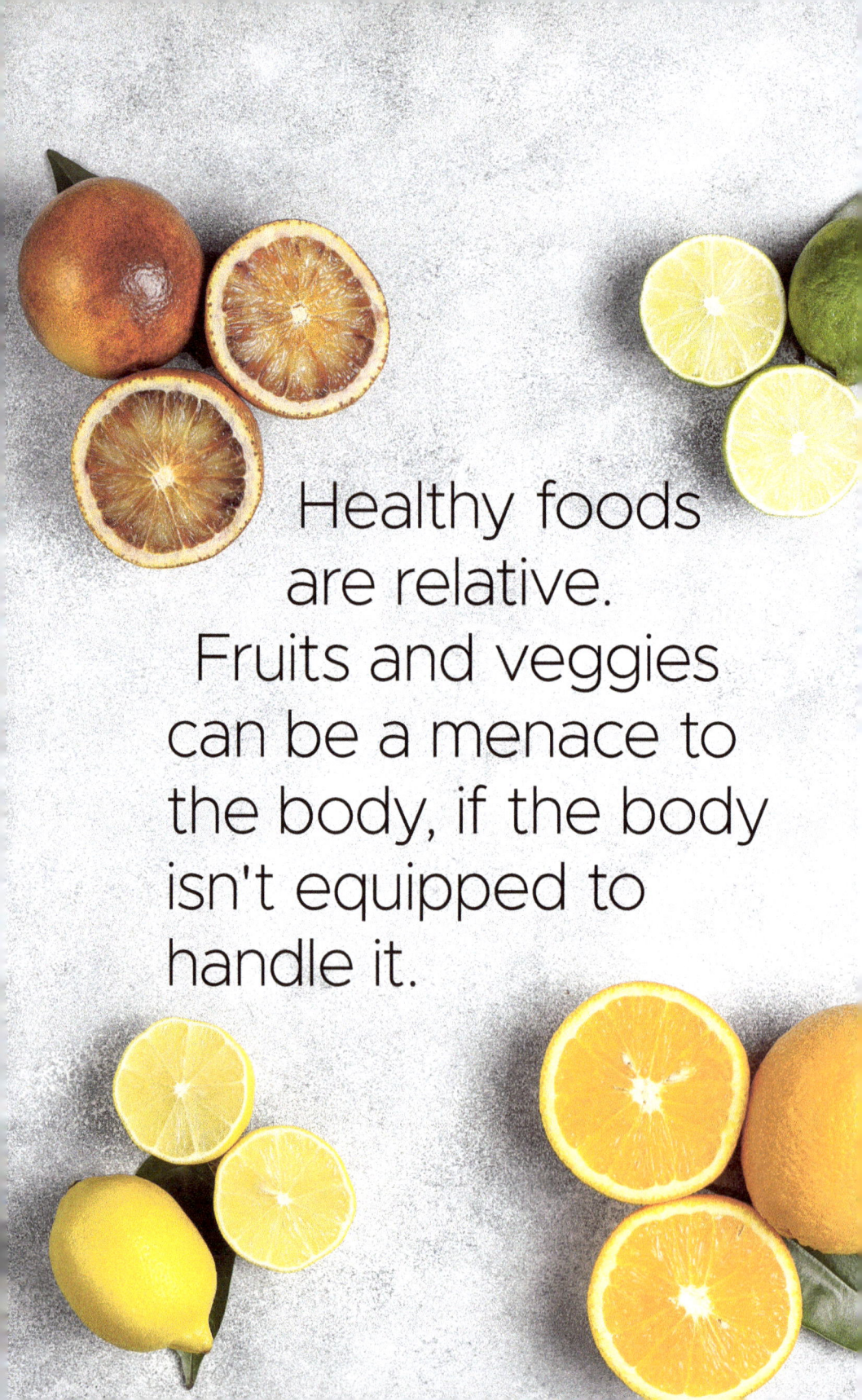

Healthy foods are relative. Fruits and veggies can be a menace to the body, if the body isn't equipped to handle it.

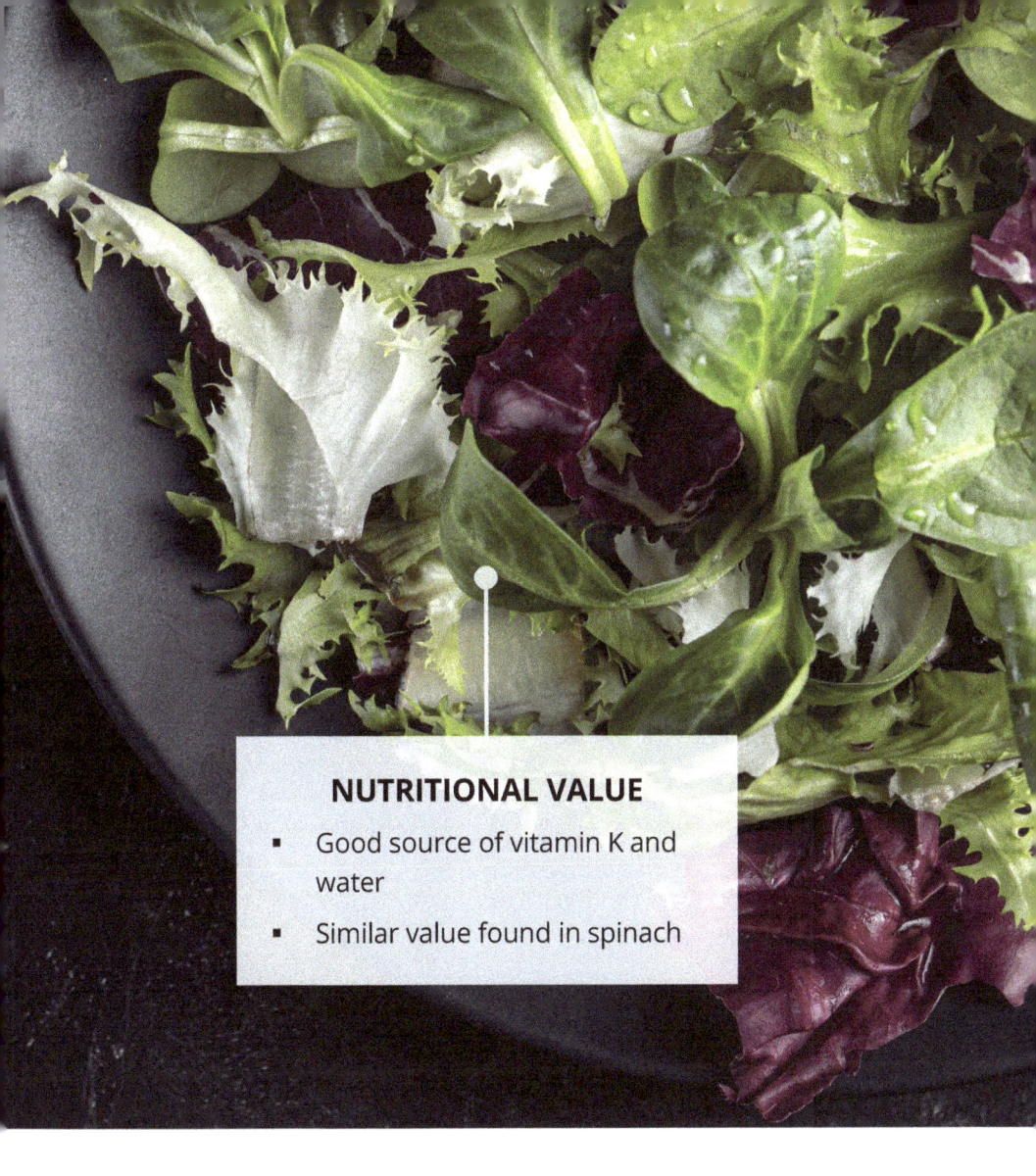

NUTRITIONAL VALUE

- Good source of vitamin K and water
- Similar value found in spinach

16 Lettuce & other Leafy Greens

Common Avoidance *Responses*

- Gas
- Bloating
- Abdominal discomfort

Food Clue *Category*

- Poor protein digestion

Food Clue *Explained*

While allergies and avoidances of lettuce and other leafy green vegetable are rare, they can be related to difficulty with the digestion of specific plant proteins (e.g., lipid transfer protein).

HEALTH CONCERNS

- Liver or gallbladder dysfunction
- Difficulty losing weight
- Chronic constipation
- Digestive conditions including irritable bowel syndrome, Crohn's disease, celiac disease

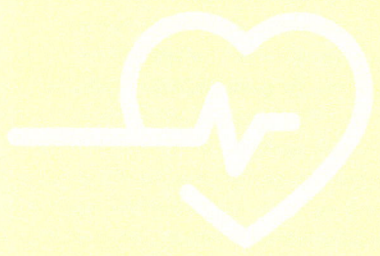

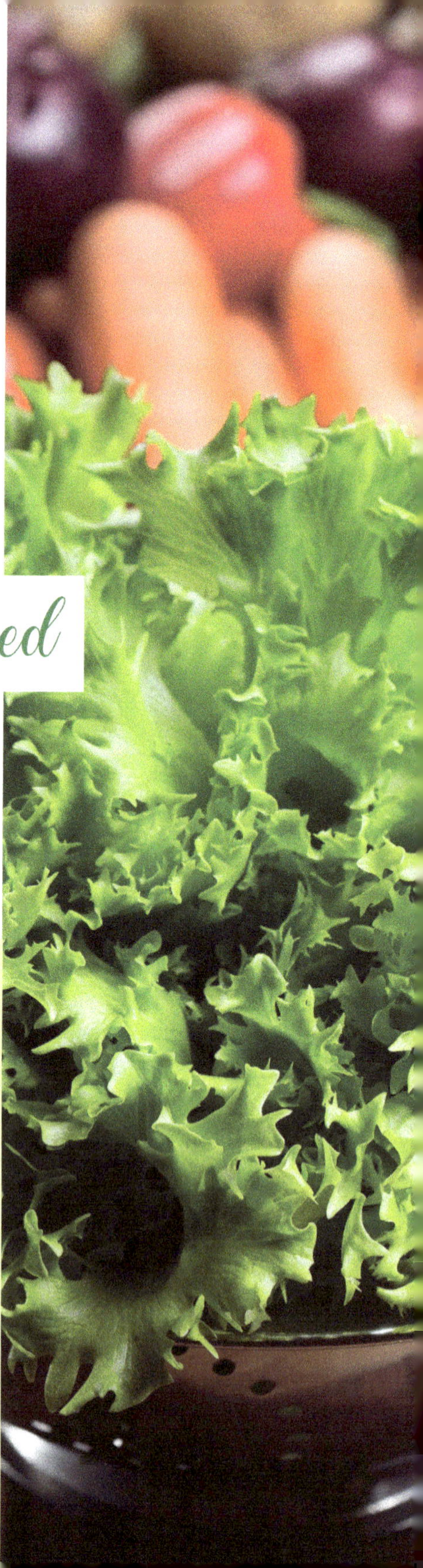

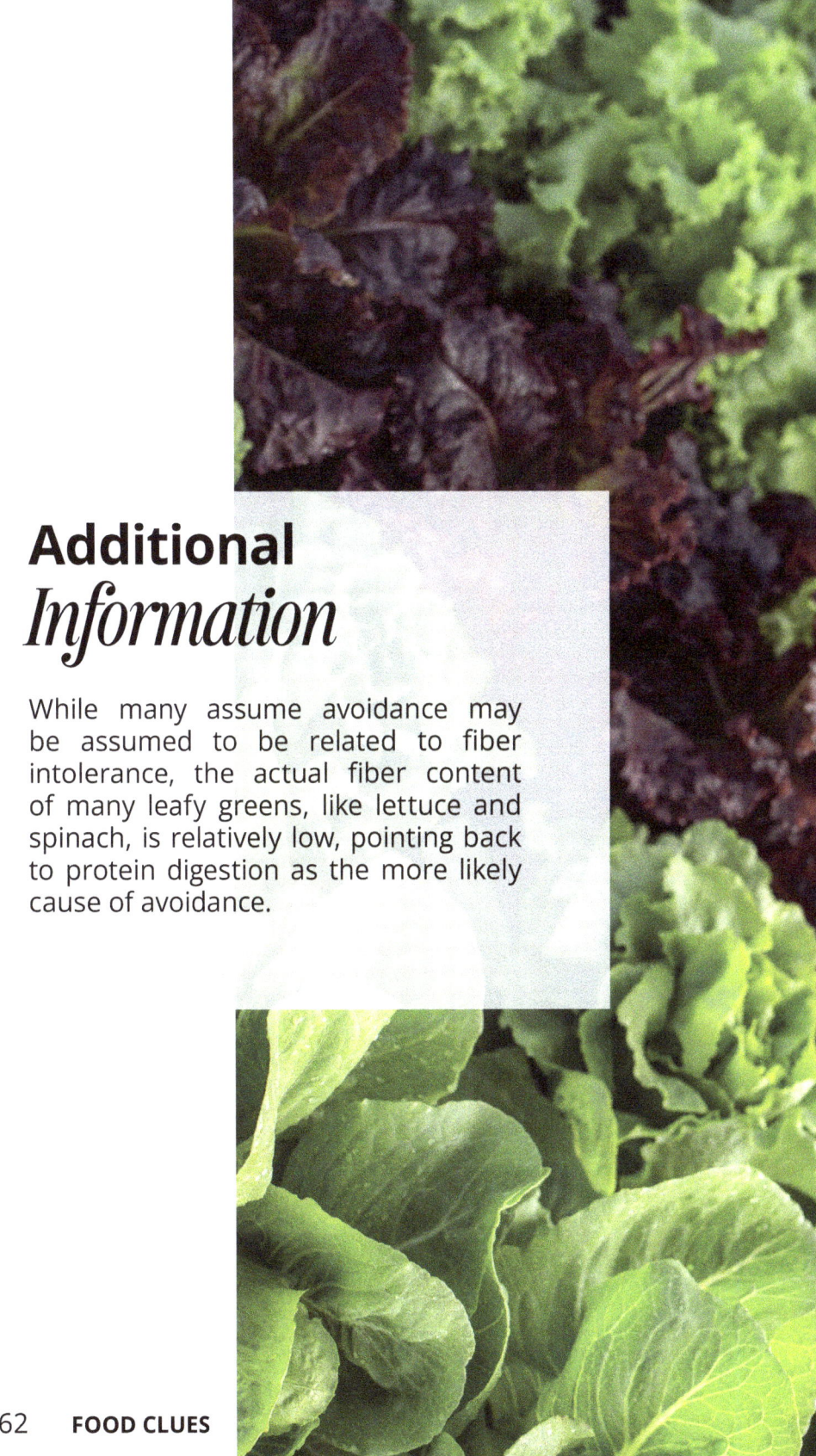

Additional
Information

While many assume avoidance may be assumed to be related to fiber intolerance, the actual fiber content of many leafy greens, like lettuce and spinach, is relatively low, pointing back to protein digestion as the more likely cause of avoidance.

Your food relationship is your body's way of talking to you.
Listen closely.

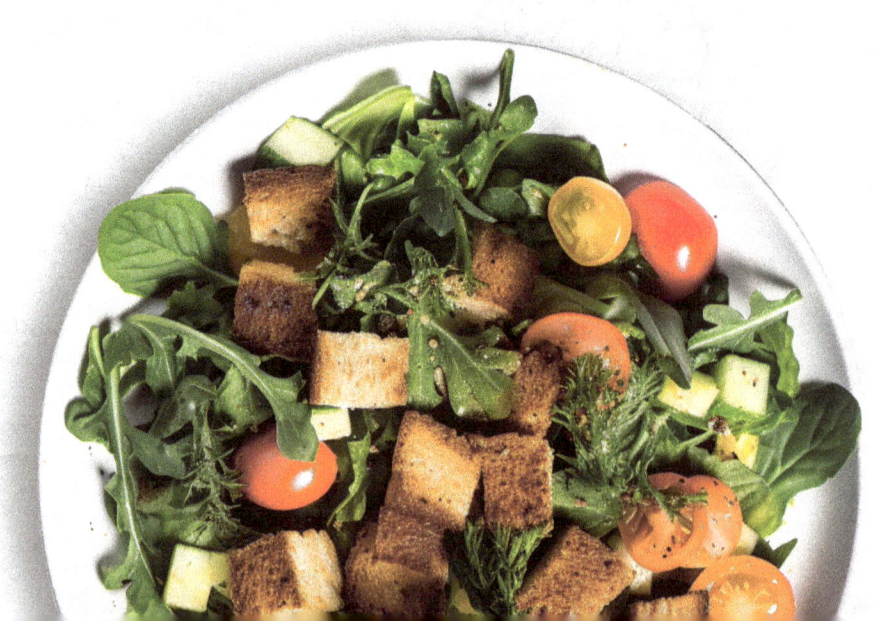

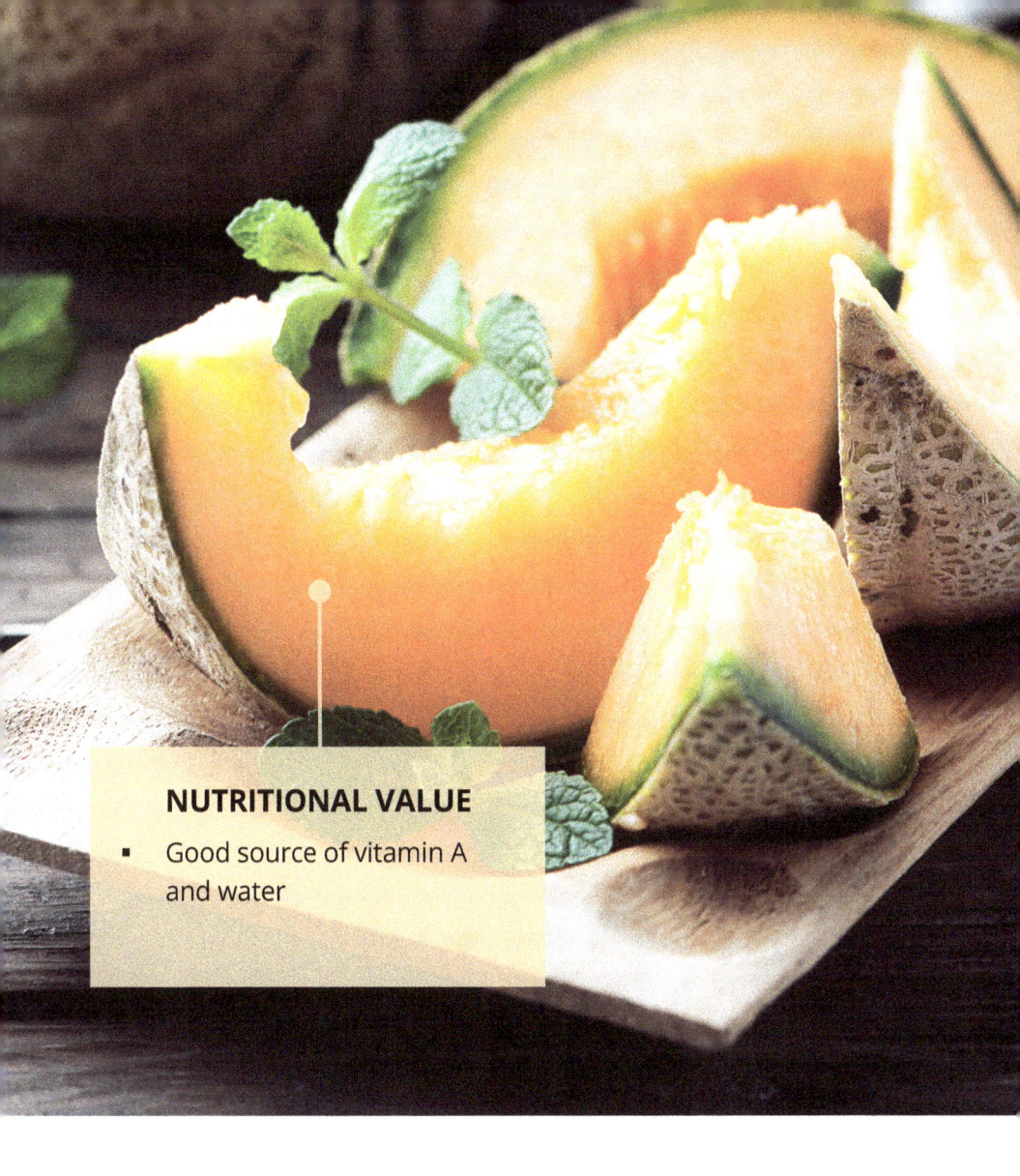

NUTRITIONAL VALUE
- Good source of vitamin A and water

17 Melon

Common Avoidance *Responses*

- Gas
- Bloating
- Abdominal discomfort
- Lip or tongue swelling
- Hives or other skin reactions

Food Clue *Category*

- Poor protein digestion

HEALTH CONCERNS
- Liver or gallbladder dysfunction
- Difficulty losing weight
- Chronic constipation
- Digestive conditions including irritable bowel syndrome, Crohn's disease, celiac disease

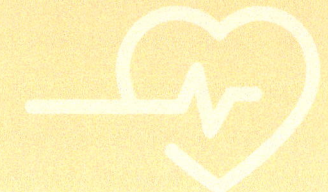

Food Clue *Explained*

Most melon reactions are related to difficulty with protein breakdown, as they have specific protein compounds in them associated with sensitivity and allergic reactions. Watermelons have only one plant protein associated with sensitivity, profilin protein. Muskmelons like honeydew and cantelope have three known plant proteins associated with sensitivity, profilin, cucumisin and PR-1.

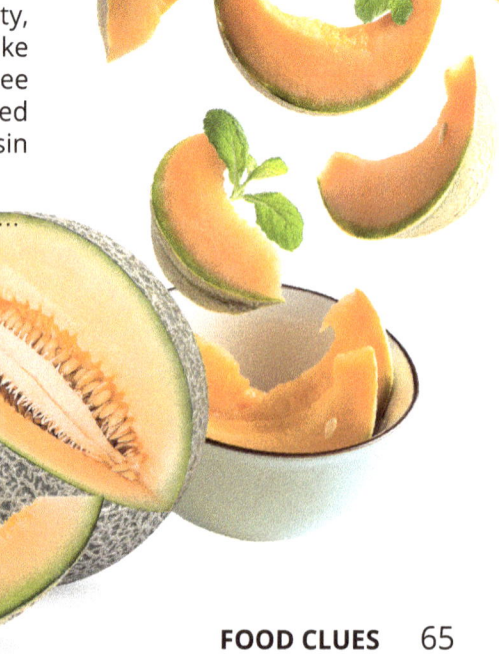

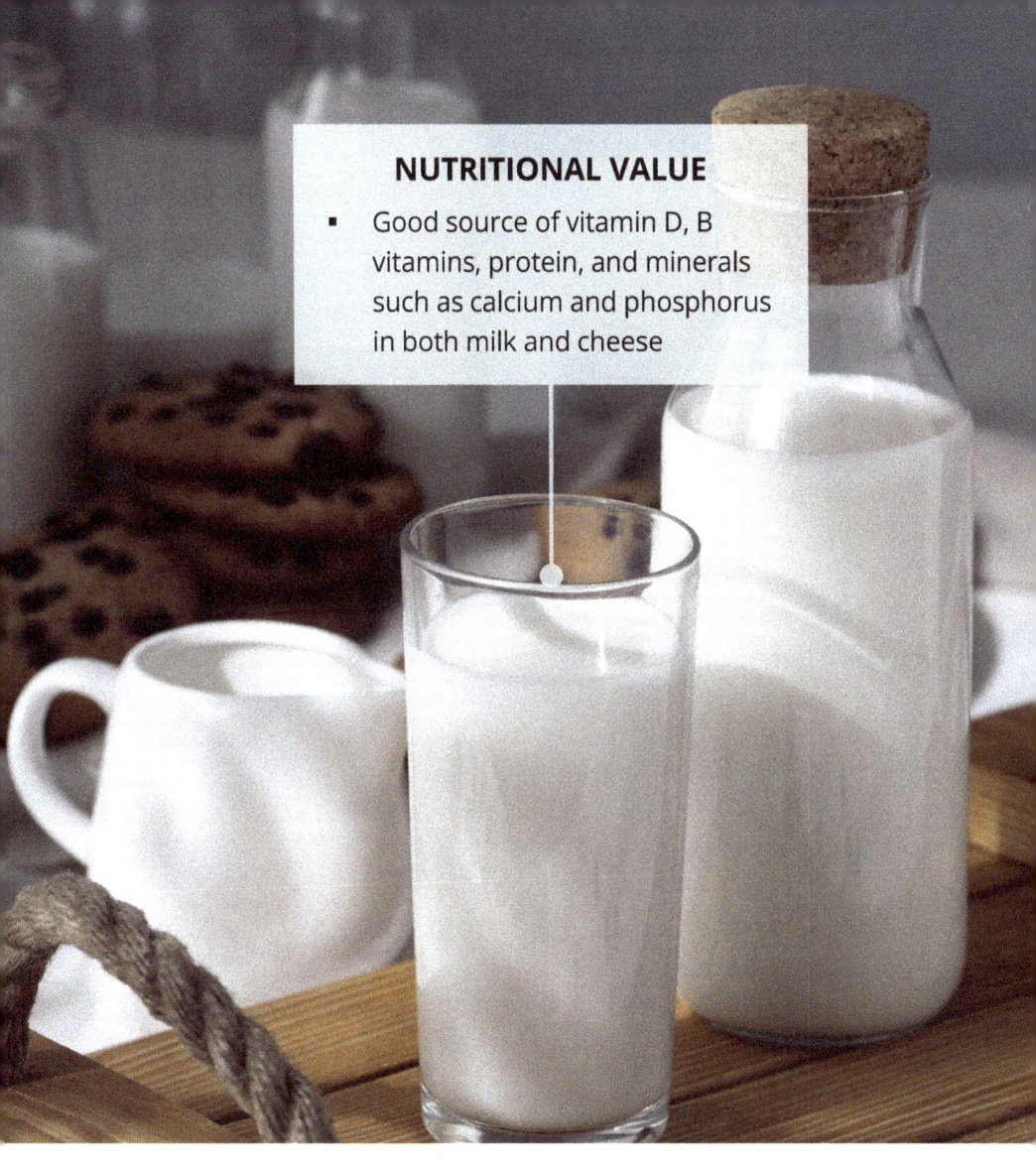

NUTRITIONAL VALUE

- Good source of vitamin D, B vitamins, protein, and minerals such as calcium and phosphorus in both milk and cheese

18 Milk

Common Avoidance *Responses*

- Gas
- Bloating
- Abdominal discomfort
- Nausea after eating or smelling
- Headache after eating or smelling
- Lip, tongue swelling
- Hives or other skin reactions

Food Clue *Category*

- Poor protein digestion
- Unbalanced gut bacteria levels

HEALTH CONCERNS

- Small intestinal bacterial overgrowth (SIBO)
- Digestive conditions including irritable bowel syndrome, Crohn's disease, celiac disease
- Emotional and mental health imbalances including anxiety, depression, autism, attention deficit disorder, attention deficit hyperactivity disorder

Food Clue *Explained*

Avoidance of dairy products is most commonly due to digestive system dysfunction.

Milk allergies are often related to difficulty with protein digestion - mainly casein and whey - which are found in milk, along with poor acid breakdown or elimination.

Lactose intolerance is related to the avoidance the glucose-based component of milk. It's likely that this avoidance response is related to elevated bacterial levels in the gut flora - as sugars are food sources for bacterias - therefore avoiding further bacterial growth by limiting its food source. High bacterial levels can cause difficulty with digestion and numerous digestive conditions..

Allergy *Stats*

- Cow's milk is considered a top allergen by the National Institute of Health.
- About 2.5% of children under age three have milk allergies, commonly based on reactions to casein and whey milk proteins and typically outgrown by adulthood.
- About 68% of the world population has lactose intolerance, avoidance of the sugar component of milk called lactose.

FOOD CLUES

Additional *Information*

Nausea or headache within the first few bites or after catching a whiff of a dairy product are also common dislike symptoms. Some people get symptoms even with the thought of eating dairy. Responses like these are more of a nervous system response, alerting you against putting something into your body that your body knows is harmful in some way.

What causes issues with dairy products?

- Inflammation within the digestive tract
- Low digestive hormones, causing poor communication between the brain and gut, making it hard for the body to know that it has proteins that it needs to break down
- Infection introduced to the body from the outside environment, disrupting normal digestive system function
- Overgrowth of bacteria in the gut to balance out existing infection and maintain gut equilibrium

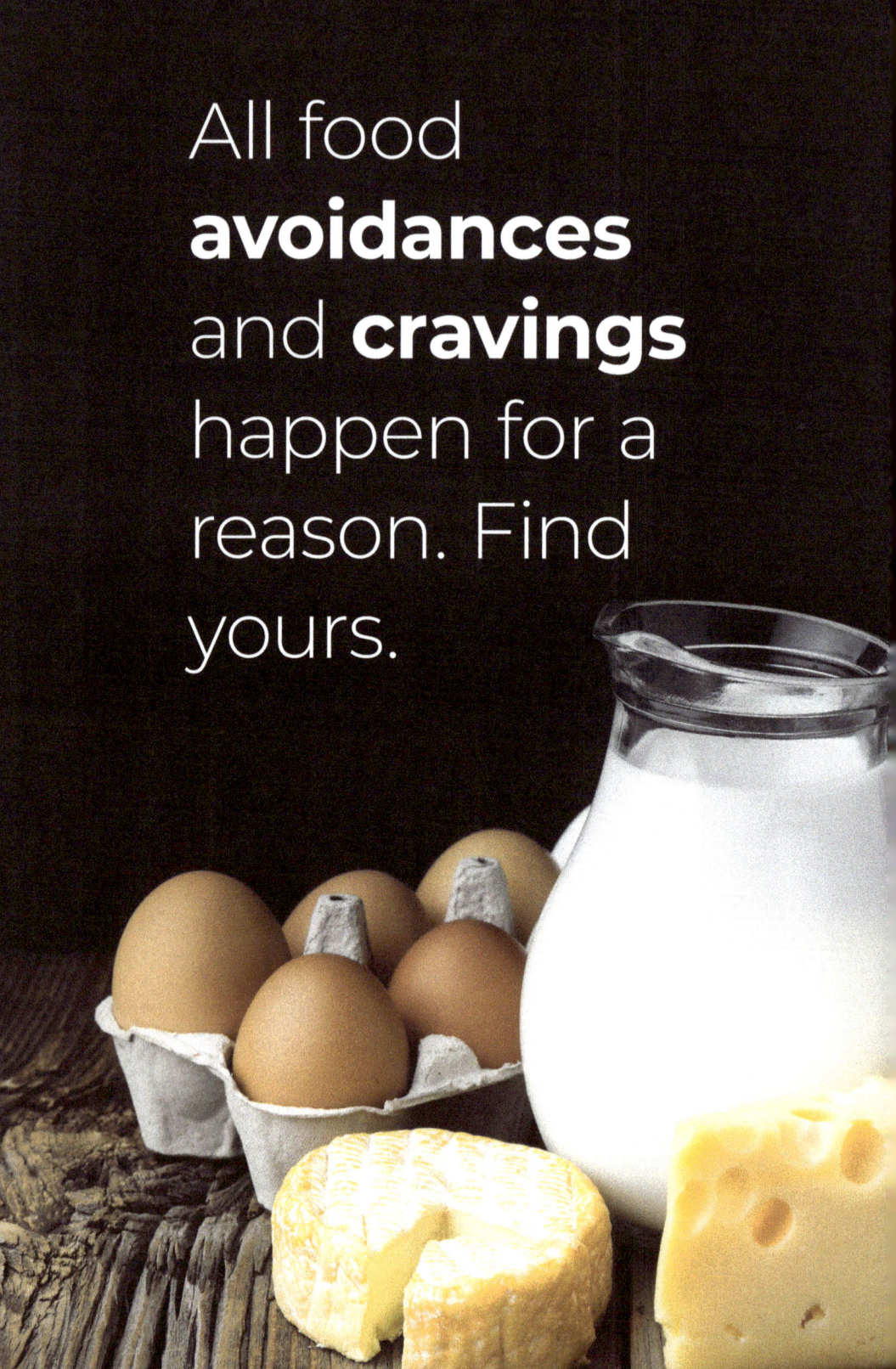

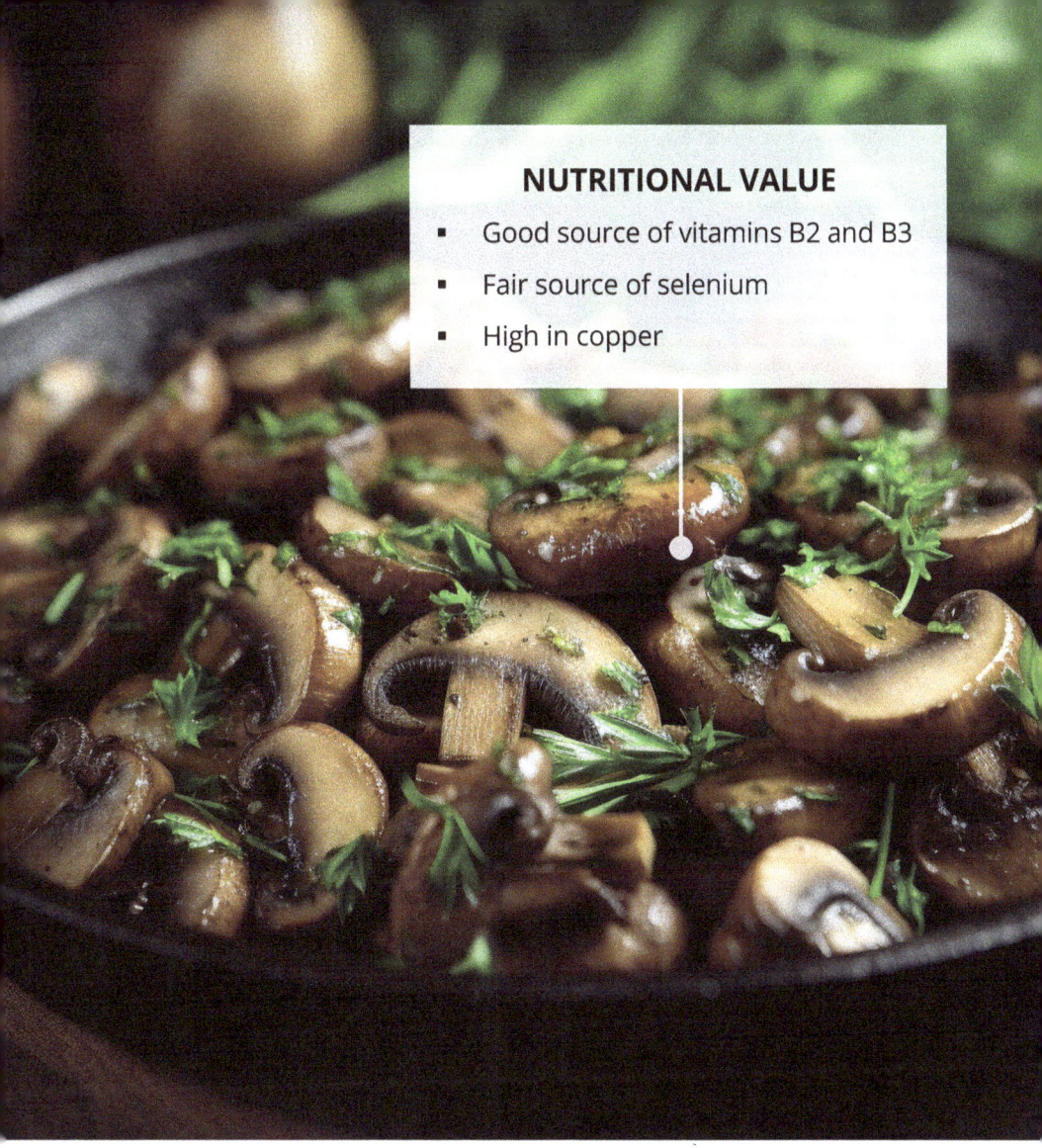

NUTRITIONAL VALUE
- Good source of vitamins B2 and B3
- Fair source of selenium
- High in copper

19 Mushrooms

Common Avoidance *Responses*

- Headache after smelling
- Nausea after smelling
- Gas
- Bloating
- Abdominal discomfort

Food Clue *Category*

- Unbalanced gut bacteria levels
- Metal toxicity
- Unbalanced immune performance

HEALTH CONCERNS

- Candida overgrowth
- Yeast infection
- Autoimmune conditions

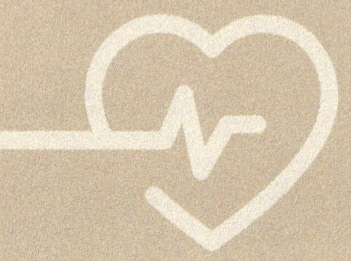

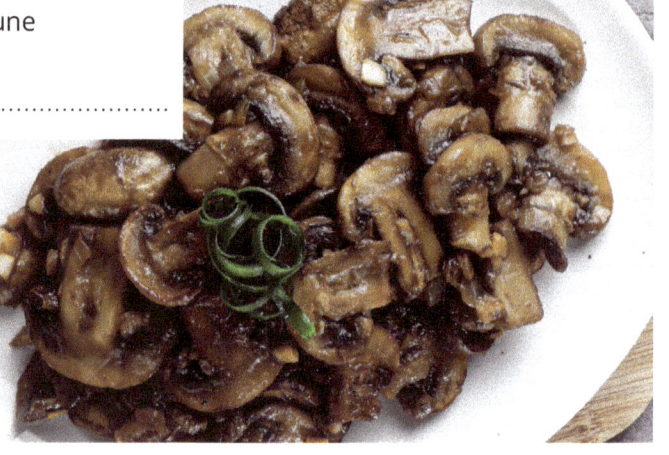

Food Clue *Explained*

Most people know that mushrooms are part of the fungus family. Many times, reactions to or avoidance of mushrooms is related to elevated fungal levels in the body.

In some cases, avoidance or reactions to mushrooms can be a sign of metal toxicity, as they are naturally high in copper. In other cases, adverse responses can indicate a poor immune response, as many mushrooms contain compounds that drive immune performance in a particular direction.

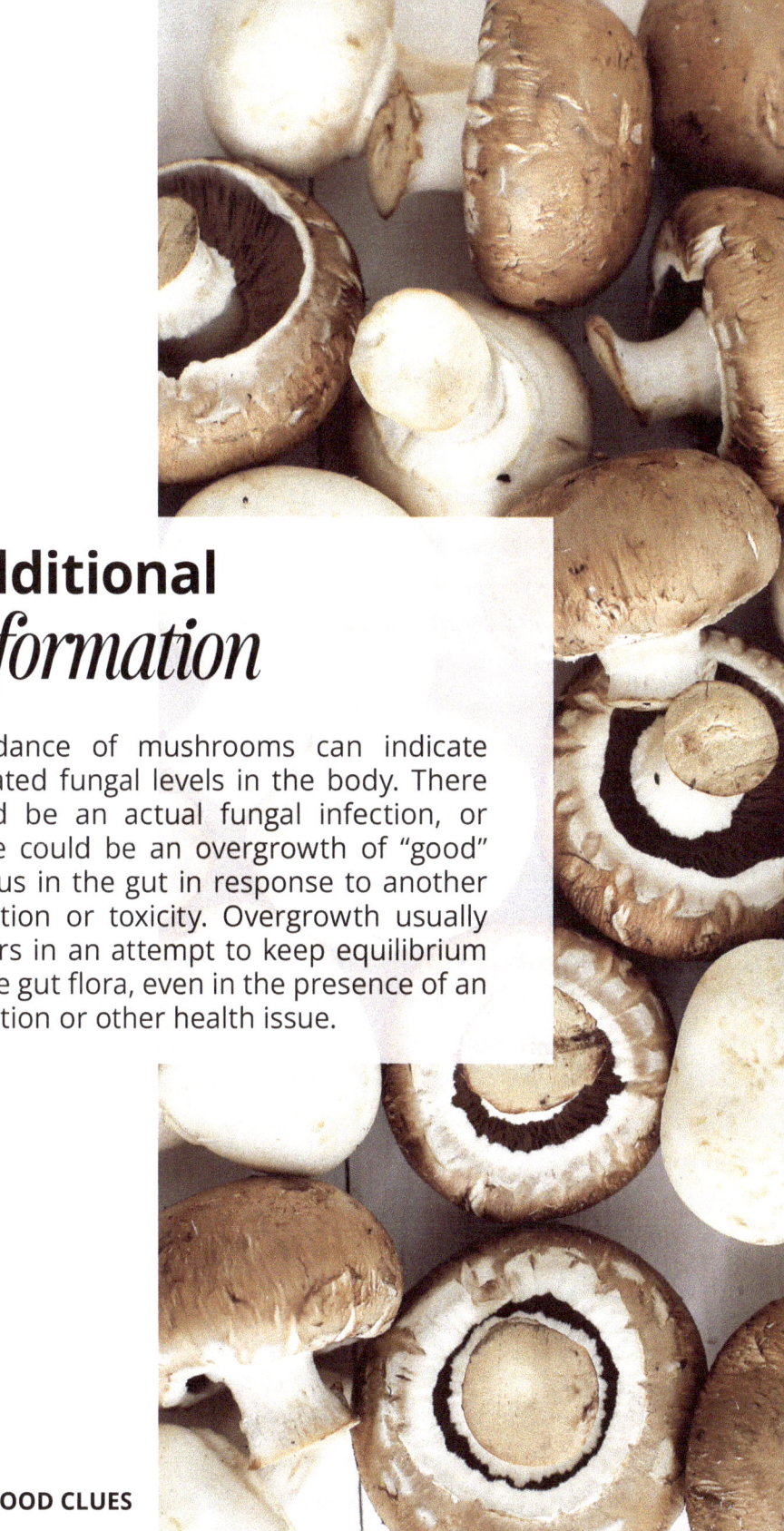

Additional
Information

Avoidance of mushrooms can indicate elevated fungal levels in the body. There could be an actual fungal infection, or there could be an overgrowth of "good" fungus in the gut in response to another infection or toxicity. Overgrowth usually occurs in an attempt to keep equilibrium in the gut flora, even in the presence of an infection or other health issue.

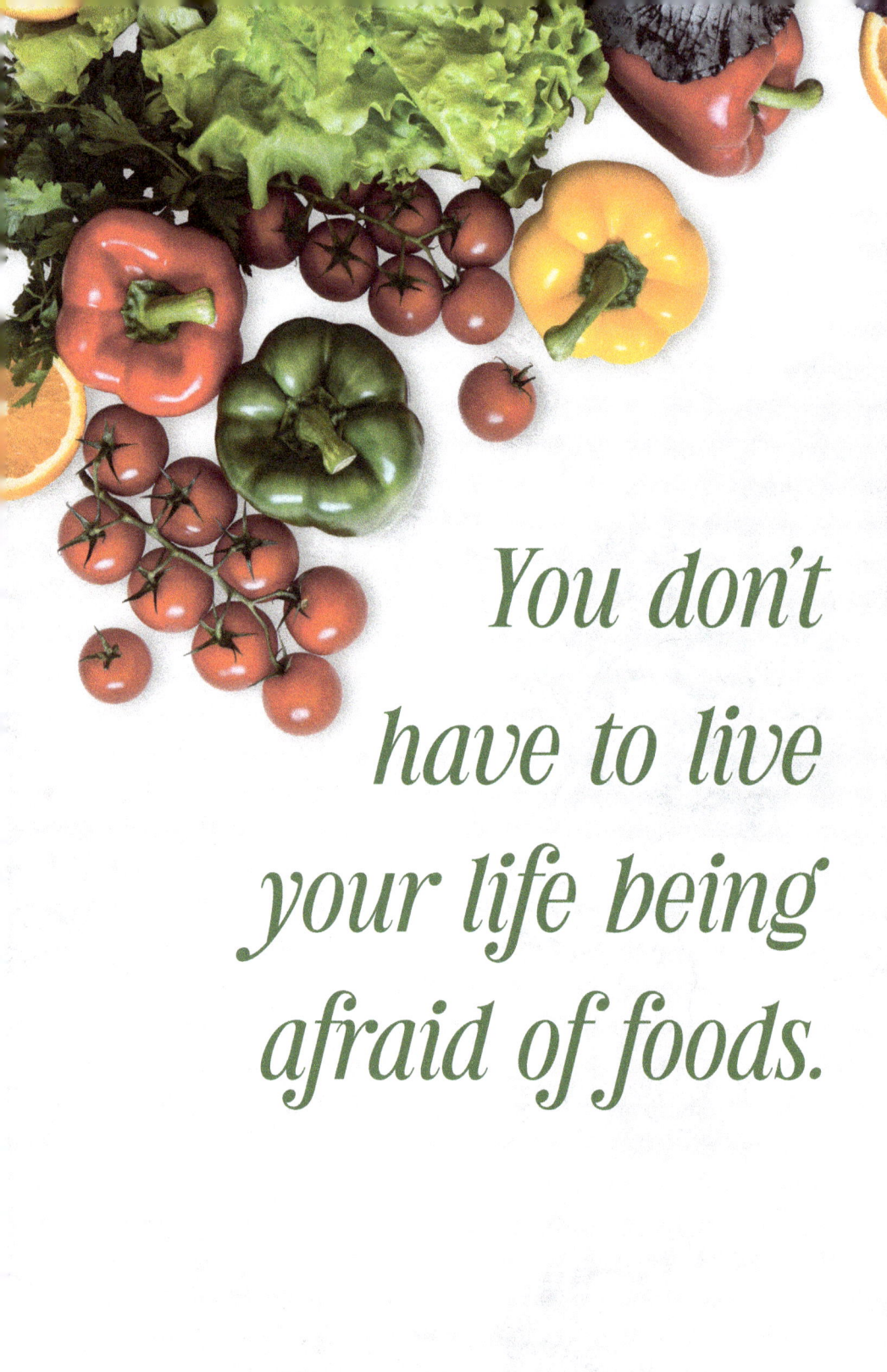

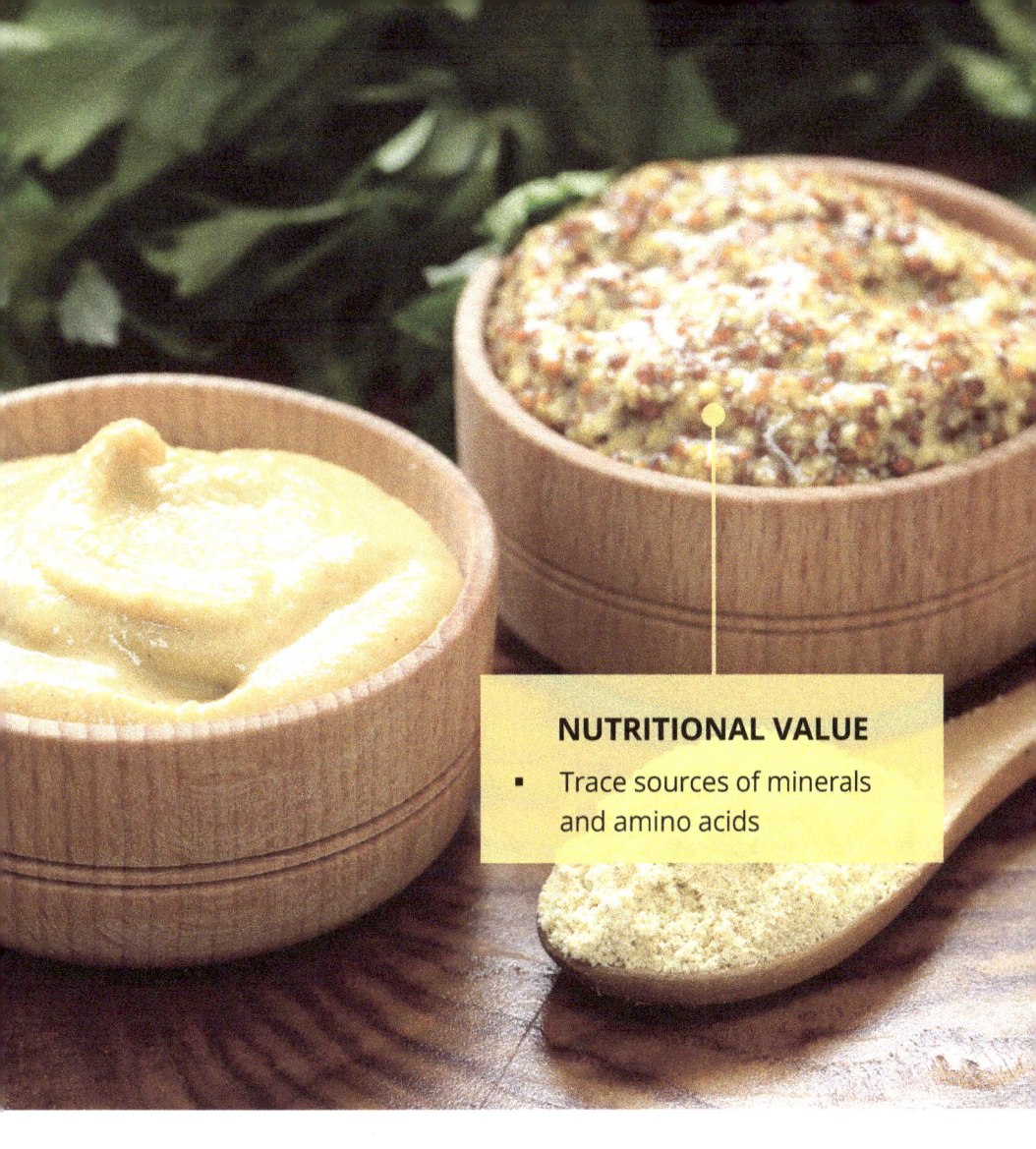

NUTRITIONAL VALUE
- Trace sources of minerals and amino acids

20 Mustard

Common Avoidance *Responses*

- Gas
- Bloating
- Indigestion
- Constipation
- Abdominal pain
- Nausea

Food Clue *Category*

- Poor protein digestion
- Poor liver function

HEALTH CONCERNS

- Liver or gallbladder dysfunction
- Small intestinal bacterial overgrowth (SIBO)
- Digestive conditions including irritable bowel syndrome, Crohn's disease, celiac disease

Food Clue *Explained*

Intolerance to mustard often signals an underlying challenge in digesting plant proteins, especially profilin. This protein is also present in pod-bearing beans like soy and peanuts. Therefore, individuals experiencing symptoms of mustard intolerance may have related soy or peanut allergies or intolerances, all likely stemming from a common issue with protein digestion.

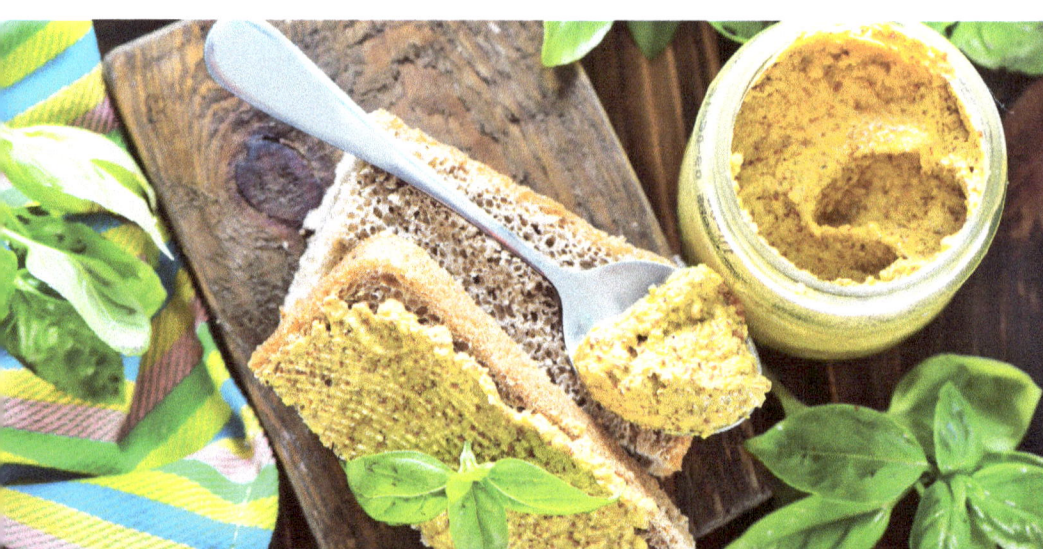

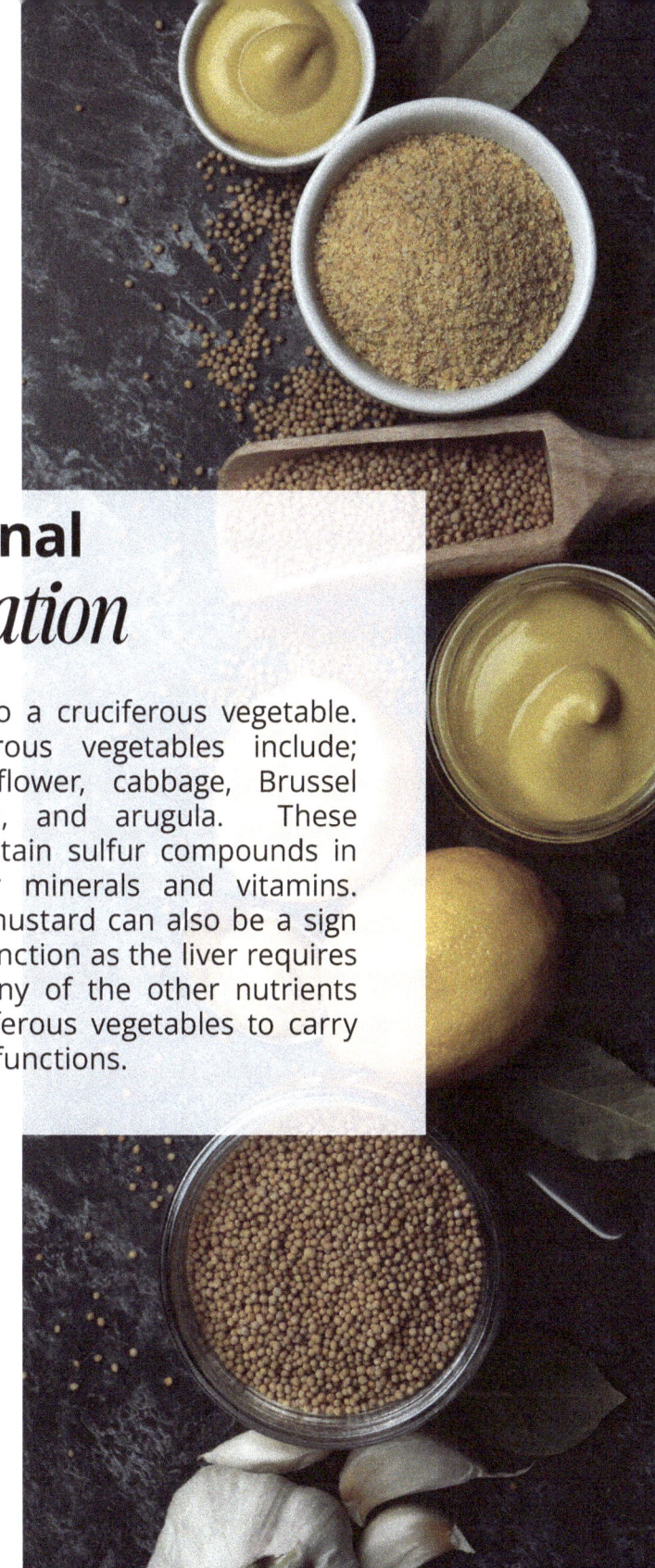

Additional
Information

Mustard is also a cruciferous vegetable. Other cruciferous vegetables include; broccoli, cauliflower, cabbage, Brussel sprout, radish, and arugula. These vegetables contain sulfur compounds in addition other minerals and vitamins. Avoidance of mustard can also be a sign of poor liver function as the liver requires sulfur and many of the other nutrients found in cruciferous vegetables to carry out numerous functions.

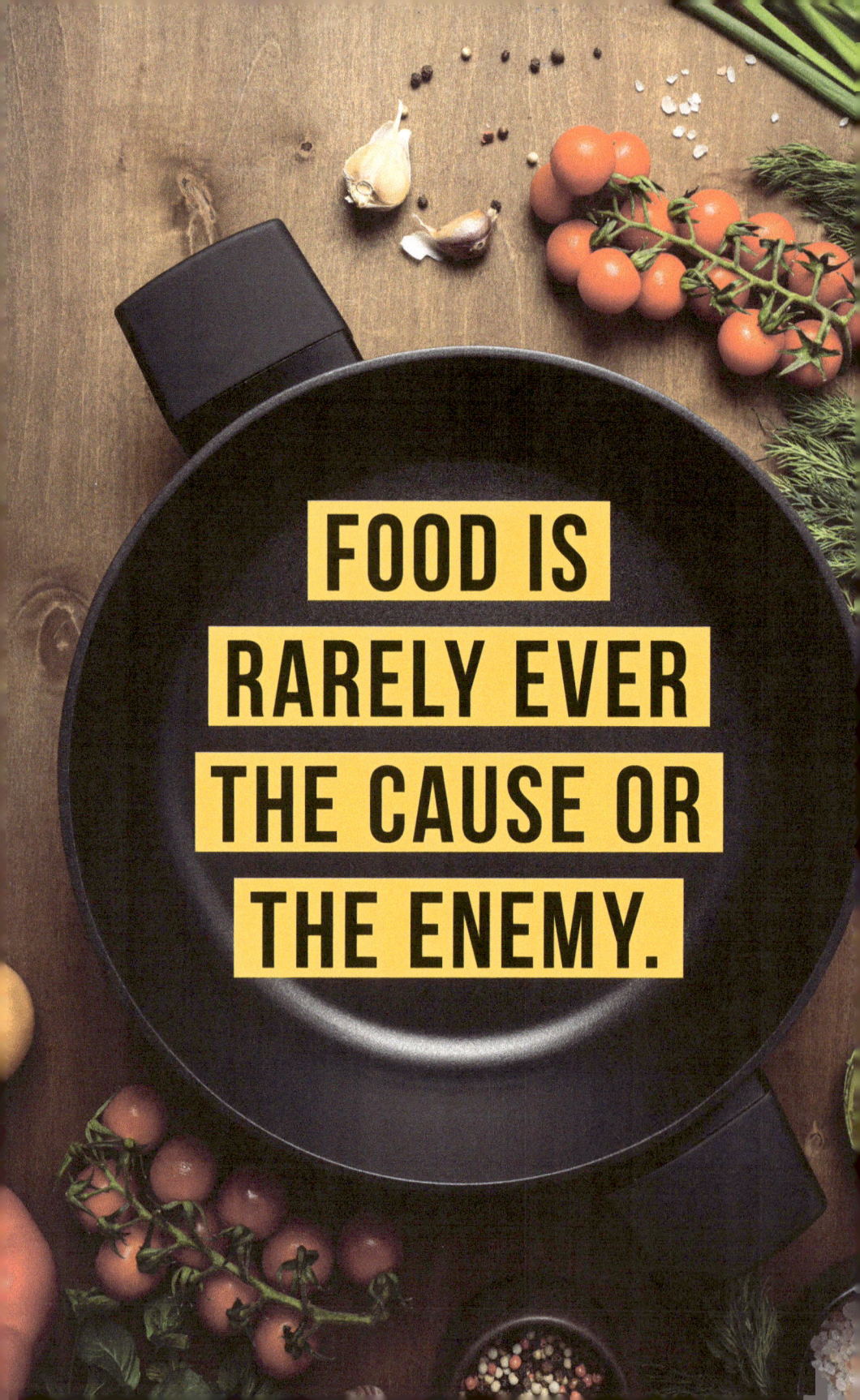

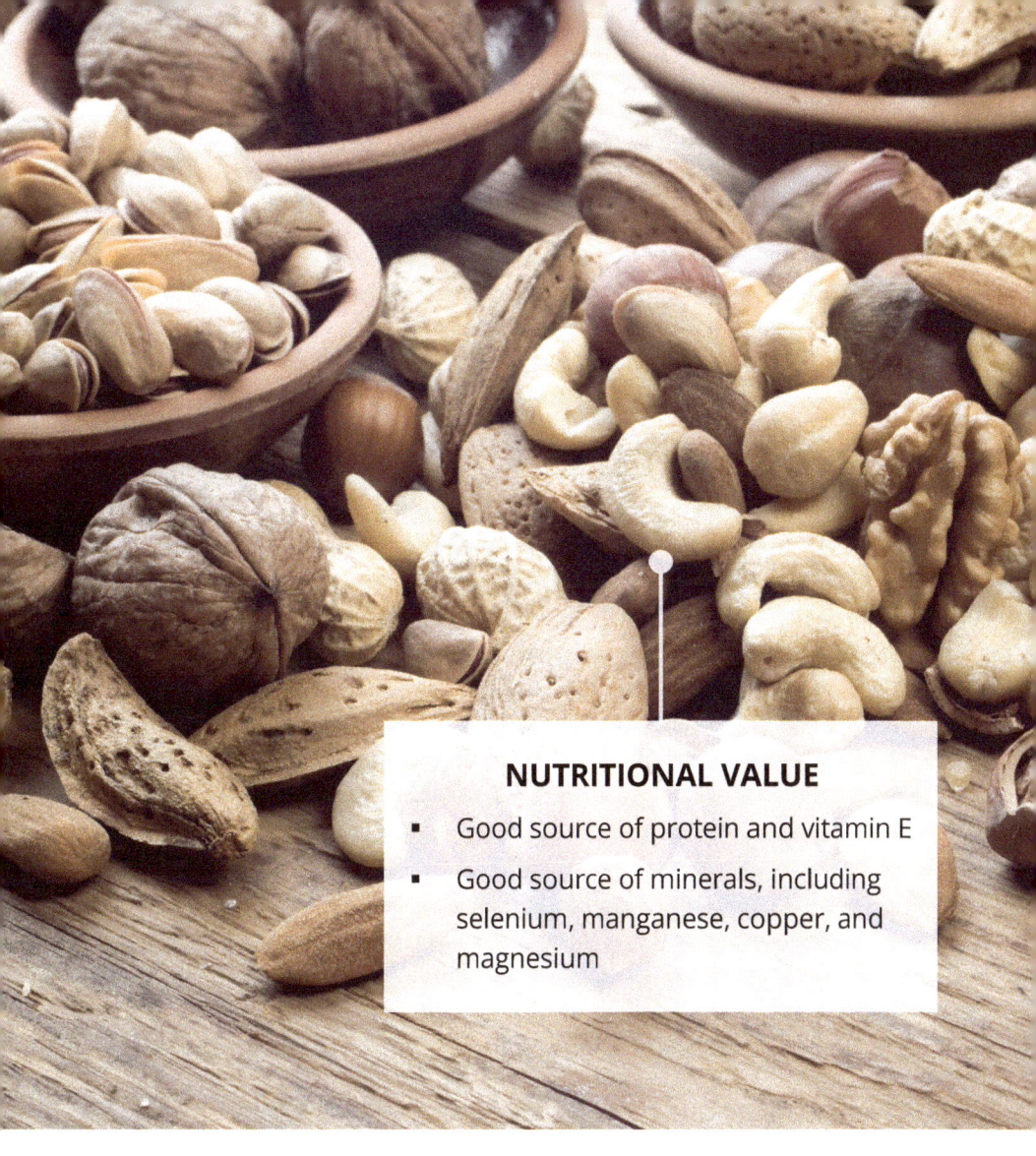

NUTRITIONAL VALUE
- Good source of protein and vitamin E
- Good source of minerals, including selenium, manganese, copper, and magnesium

21 Nuts

Common Avoidance *Responses*

- Lip or tongue swelling
- Itchy skin
- Gas, bloating, or nausea
- Anaphylactic responses in extreme cases

Food Clue *Category*

- Fatty acid imbalance
- Unbalanced gut bacteria levels

Food Clue *Explained*

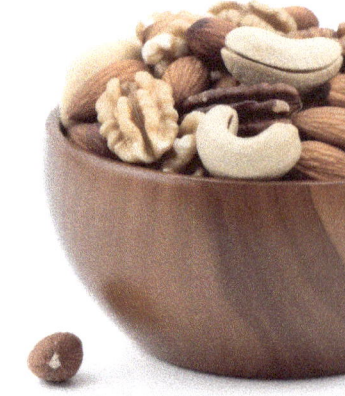

Much like avocados, nut reactions can suggest an imbalance in omega-6 and omega-3 fatty acids. Typically, the body thrives with a ratio of omega-6 to omega-3 levels closer to 3:1.

Allergy *Stats*

- Tree nuts include nuts such as walnuts, almonds, pecans, cashews and more
- Tree nuts are considered a top allergen by the National Institute of Health
- Tree nut allergies affect roughly 0.5 to 1% of the U.S. population

HEALTH CONCERNS

- Small intestinal bacterial overgrowth (SIBO)
- Estrogen imbalance
- Menstrual cycle dysfunction or conditions including heavy bleeding, missed cycles, endometriosis, and polycystic ovary syndrome (PCOS)
- Digestive conditions including irritable bowel syndrome, Crohn's disease, celiac disease
- Emotional and mental health imbalances including anxiety, depression, autism, attention deficit disorder, attention deficit hyperactivity disorder

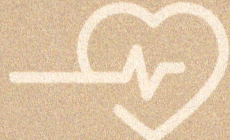

Additional
Information

A common reason for fatty acid imbalance can be an unhealthy diet, particularly one that includes high levels of processed foods, which often have much higher levels of omega-6 than omega-3 fatty acids. Research has shown that diets high in processed foods, which are common in the United States, can have omega-6 to omega-3 ratios up to five times the normal ratio.

Diets high in omega-6 fatty acids can increase inflammatory cell performance and break down the intestinal lining, also known as "leaky gut." This can allow toxins and germs to escape through the thin lining into the bloodstream, travel to other areas of the body and set the stage for organ dysfunction and system illness or disease.

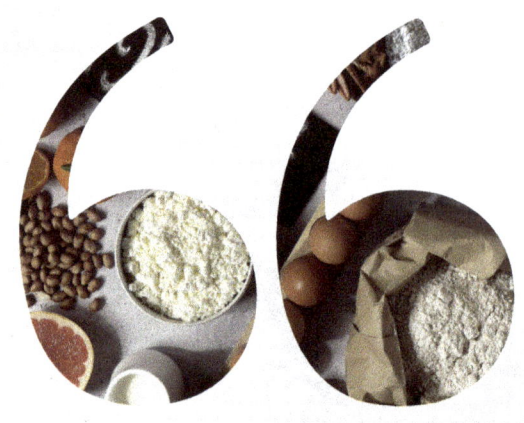

Food *allergies* are hurdles, not roadblocks.

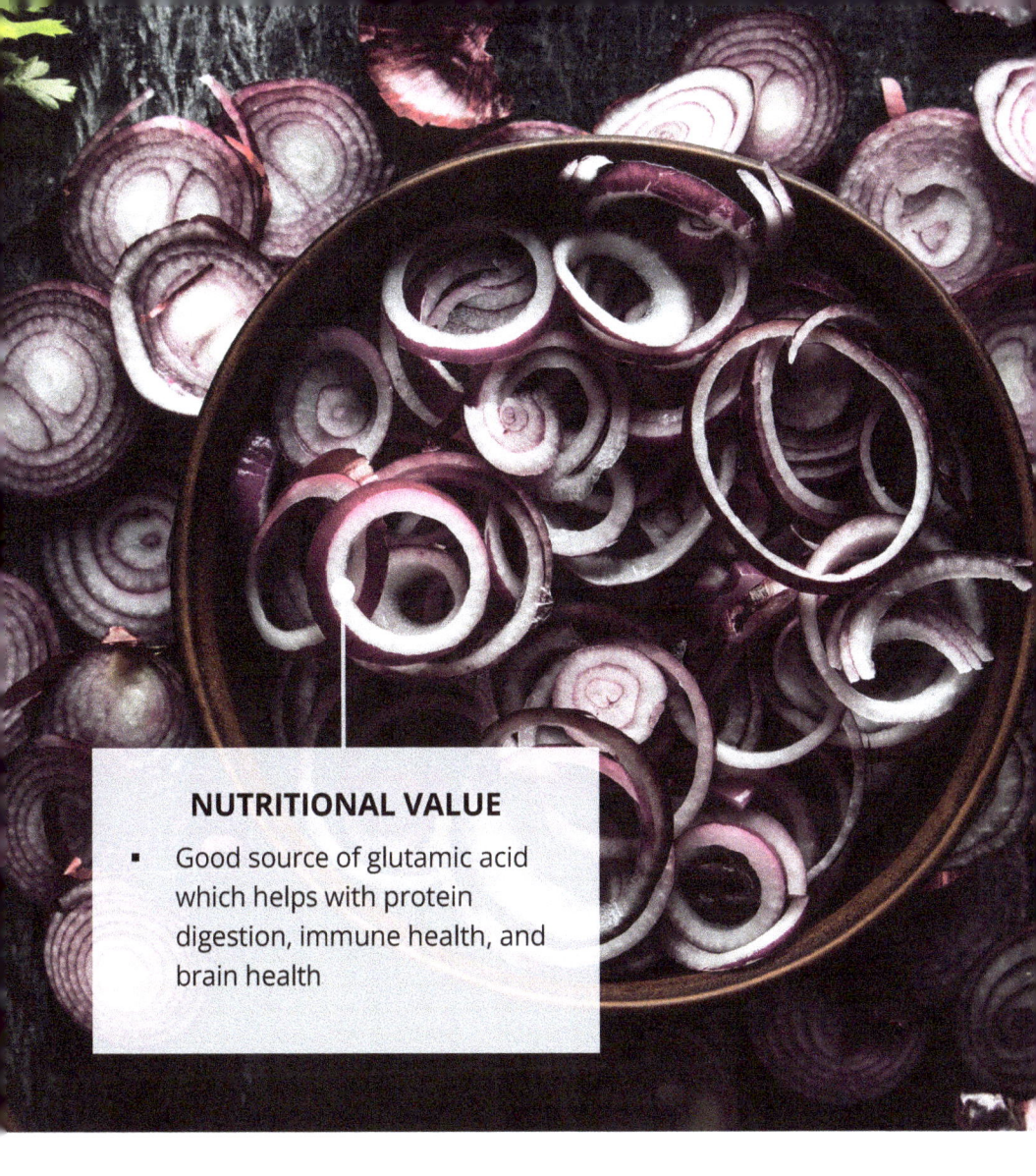

NUTRITIONAL VALUE

- Good source of glutamic acid which helps with protein digestion, immune health, and brain health

22 Onions

Common Avoidance *Responses*

- Gas
- Bloating
- Abdominal discomfort

Food Clue *Category*

- Unbalanced immune performance

HEALTH CONCERNS

- Autoimmune conditions
- Liver or gallbladder dysfunction
- Mast cell activation syndrome

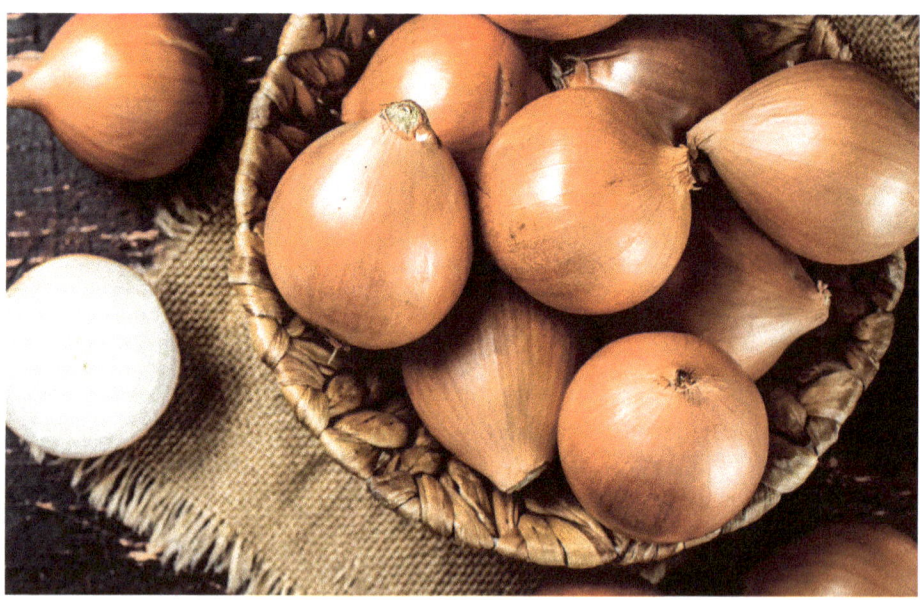

Food Clue *Explained*

A common cause of onion reactions is elevated histamine levels in the body. Histamines stimulate stomach acid secretion, help to reduce inflammation, dilate blood vessels, support muscle contractions in the intestines and lungs, and influence heart rate. If any of the other organs or systems driving those functions become impaired, histamine levels may be boosted as compensation to keep those functions going.

Additional *Information*

Tearing of the eyes when cutting onions is often a response to histamine levels in the body. Have you ever noticed that sometimes your eyes tear up when cutting onions and sometimes they don't? They usually tear up when histamine levels are too high in your body.

Two key drivers behind heightened histamine levels and onion avoidance are infection and particularly toxicity. Whether from the accumulation of either over time or the acquisition of a new ones as another is eliminated, unresolved infections and toxins are key factors in elevating histamine levels.

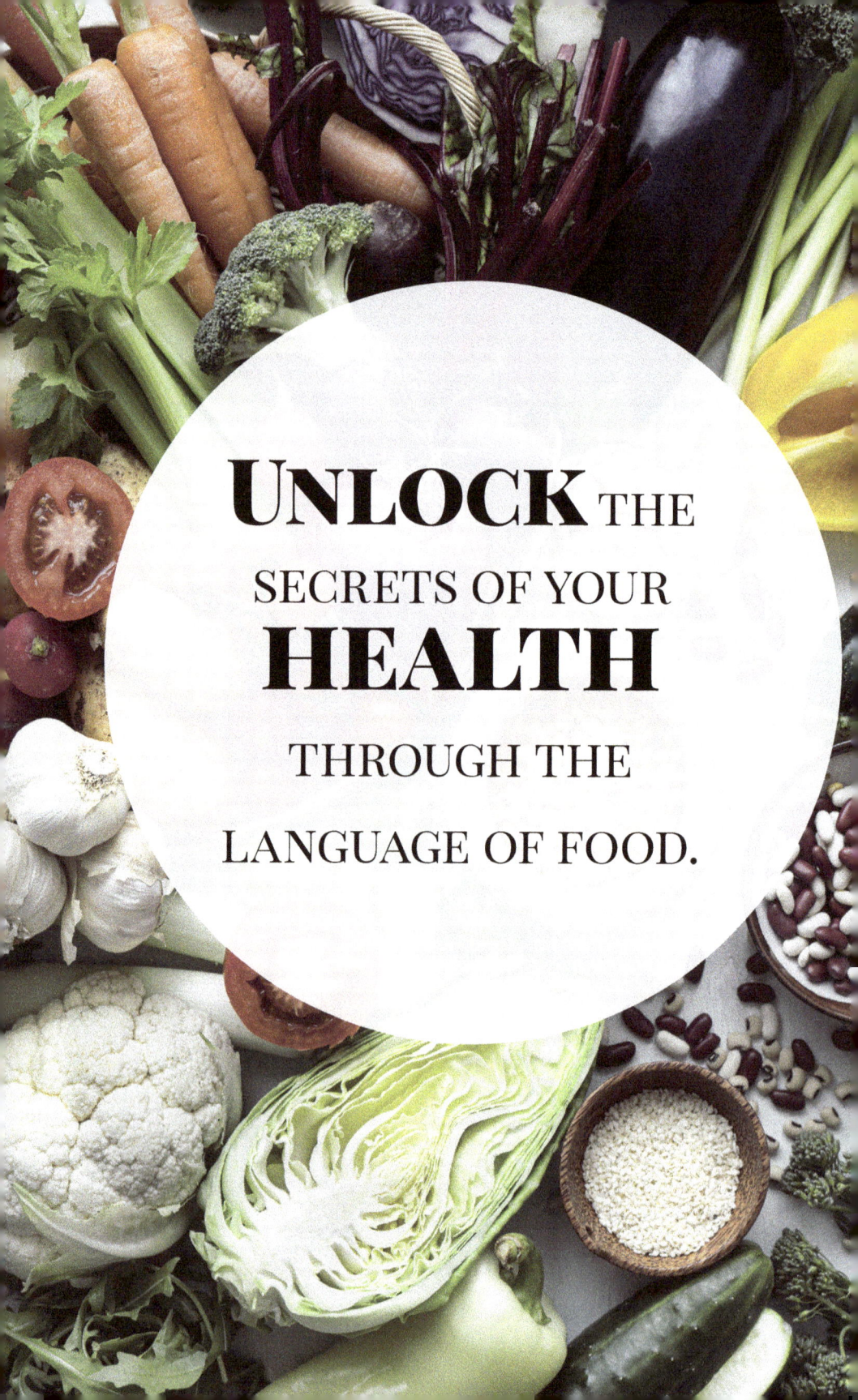

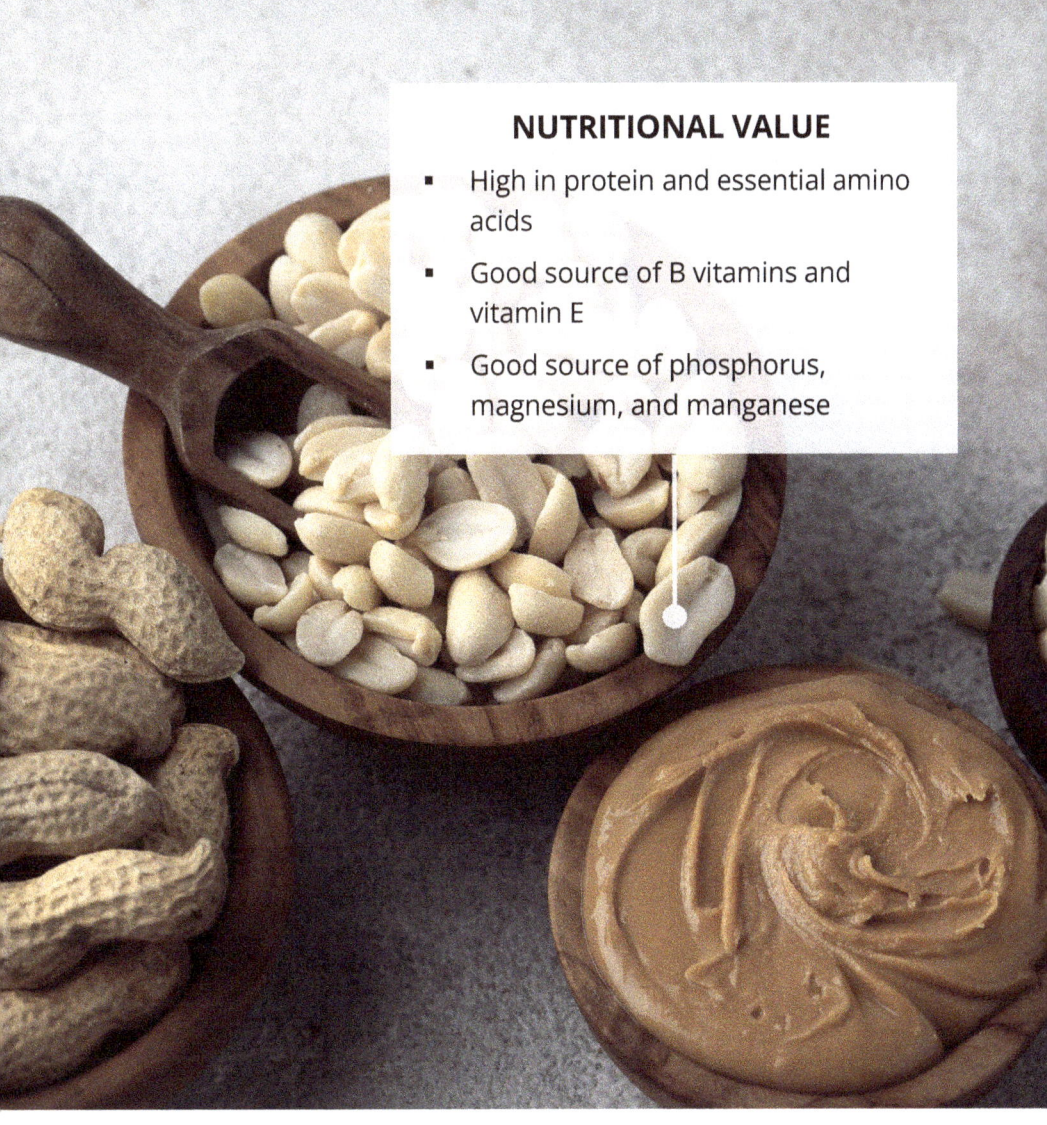

NUTRITIONAL VALUE

- High in protein and essential amino acids
- Good source of B vitamins and vitamin E
- Good source of phosphorus, magnesium, and manganese

23 Peanuts

Common Avoidance *Responses*

- Headache or nausea after smelling
- Lip or tongue swelling
- Itchy skin
- Gas, bloating, or nausea
- Anaphylactic responses in extreme cases

Food Clue *Category*

- Fatty acid imbalance
- Poor protein digestion
- Poor acid management

HEALTH CONCERNS

- Digestive conditions including irritable bowel syndrome, Crohn's disease, celiac disease
- Emotional and mental health imbalances including anxiety, depression, autism, attention deficit disorder, attention deficit hyperactivity disorder
- Autoimmune conditions including lupus, scleroderma, fibromyalgia and thyroid dysfunction

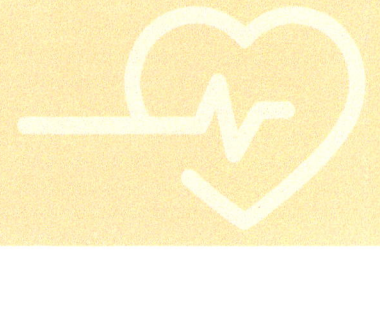

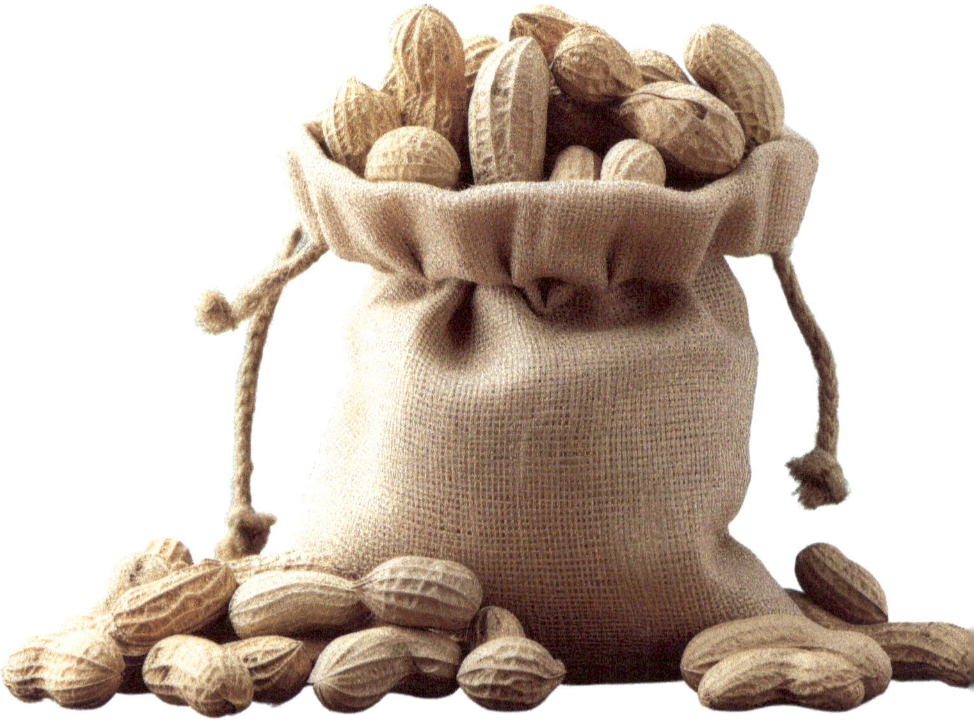

Food Clue *Explained*

Similar to many tree nuts, peanuts have a high omega-6 to omega-3 ratio. Foods high in omega-6 fatty acids can increase inflammatory cell performance and break down the intestinal lining, also known as 'leaky gut' This can allow toxins and germs to escape through the thin lining into the bloodstream, travel to other areas of the body and set the stage for organ dysfunction and system illness or disease.

Additionally, since peanuts are high in fat and protein, it also means that they are considerably acidic, as fats breakdown to fatty acids and proteins break down to amino acids. Therefore it's likely that peanut allergies could be an indicator of poor acid management in the body.

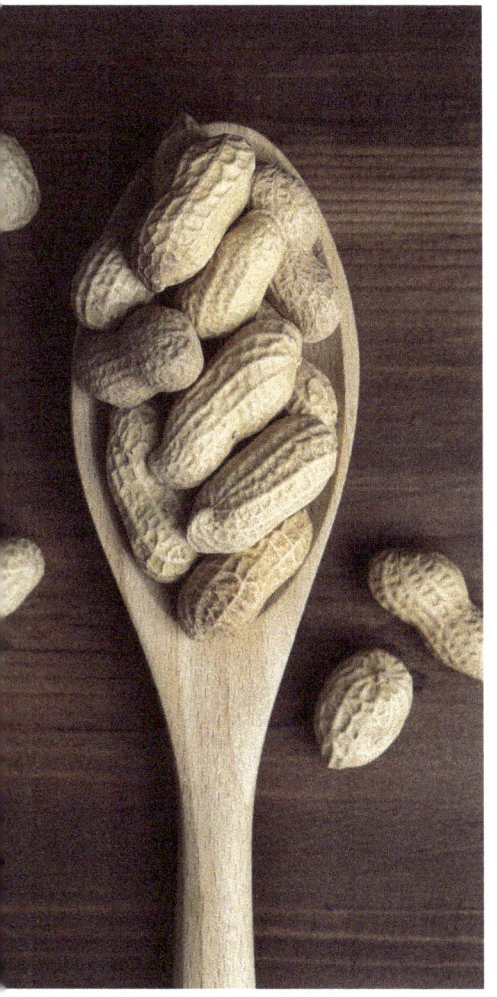

Allergy *Stats*

- Sprouted peanuts are grown in the ground, which are part of the legume family, are more similar to beans than tree nuts in characteristics
- Peanuts are considered a top allergen by the National Institute of Health
- Peanut allergies affect about 2% of the general population in Western territories (increased from 1% in earlier studies)
- Recent US studies revealed about 1% of adults report having a peanut or tree nut allergy, and about 2% of children

Additional *Information*

Poor acid management often results in poor acid elimination. Unlike carbs, sugars, and some vitamins and minerals, the human body has little to no capacity to store excess acids and many acidic compounds are supposed to be used and the excess eliminated. If excess acids aren't properly eliminated the backup can cause body performance issues but more importantly the body will protect itself by utilizing avoidance or protective mechanisms to prevent you from ingesting more acids that it can't process likely resulting in the allergic response.

It's likely that anaphylaxis is a severe response to an extremely significant acid management issue; a key cell that recognizes problematic substances in the body (IgE) may be excessively released in an excessive attempt to prevent the introduction of more acid based substances into the body.

There are numerous aspects of acid management to consider - acid breakdown, neutralization, conversion, transport, absorption, usage and elimination to name a few - the number and severity of these management issues likely explains why degrees of sensitivity can vary, spanning from nausea when smelled all the way to emergent anaphylaxis.

Knowing that a natural protective mechanism of the body is to avoid substances that threaten it's performance or safety, rejections of peanuts can be proportional to the degree of difficulty managing fats, proteins or their acidic components.

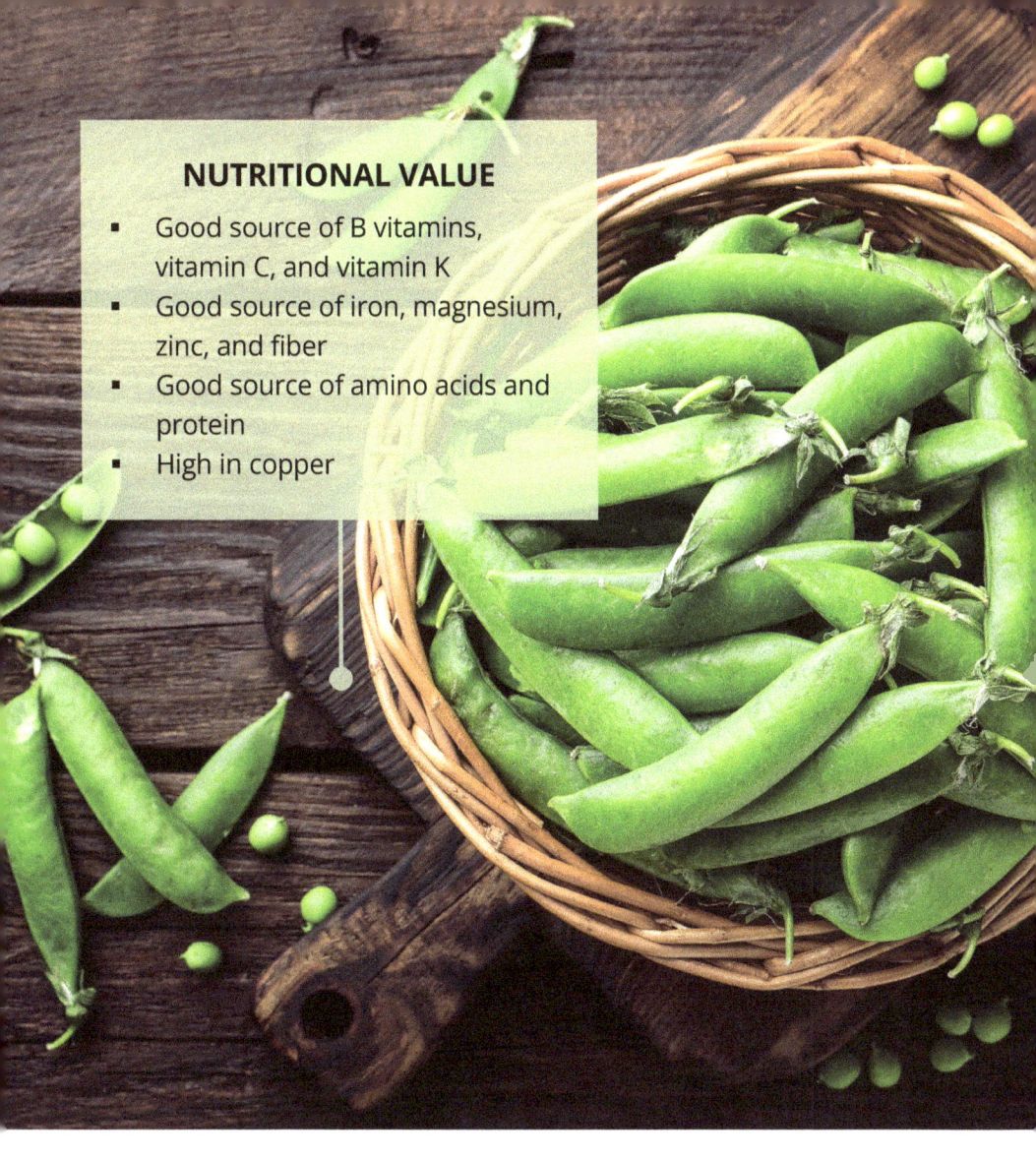

NUTRITIONAL VALUE

- Good source of B vitamins, vitamin C, and vitamin K
- Good source of iron, magnesium, zinc, and fiber
- Good source of amino acids and protein
- High in copper

24 Peas

Common Avoidance *Responses*

- Gas
- Bloating
- Indigestion
- Constipation
- Abdominal pain
- Nausea

Food Clue *Category*

- Poor protein digestion

HEALTH CONCERNS

- Small intestinal bacterial overgrowth (SIBO)
- Digestive conditions including irritable bowel syndrome, Crohn's disease, celiac disease

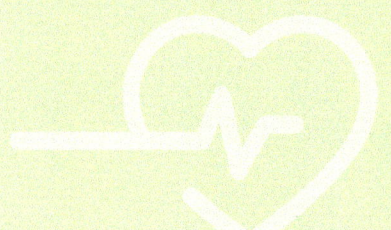

Food Clue *Explained*

Intolerance to peas is often a sign of difficulty with digesting proteins, including those specific to beans that come in pods, like soybeans and peanuts. Reactions are often related to the complexity of the protein compounds in the bean, so you can have reactions to some beans but not others.

Additional *Information*

A common cause for sensitivity to peas tends to be SIBO, small intestinal bacterial overgrowth, which disrupts the delicate balance of bacteria in the gut, creates inflammation, and makes digestion difficult.

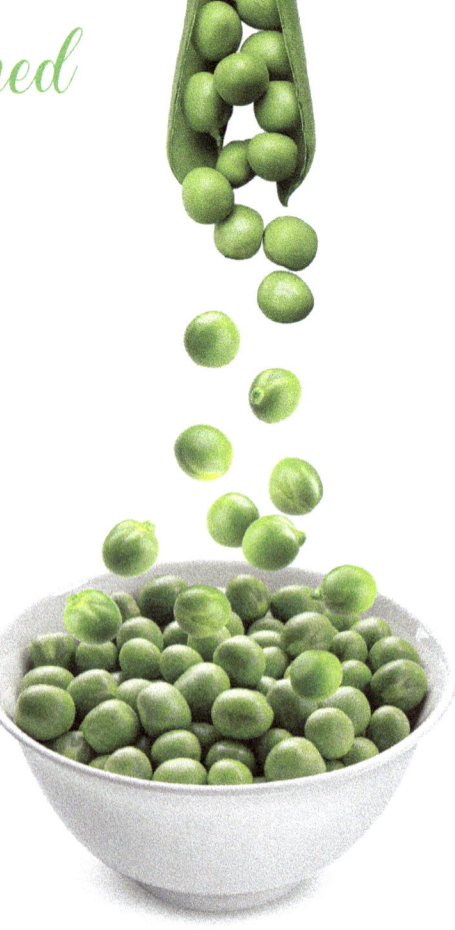

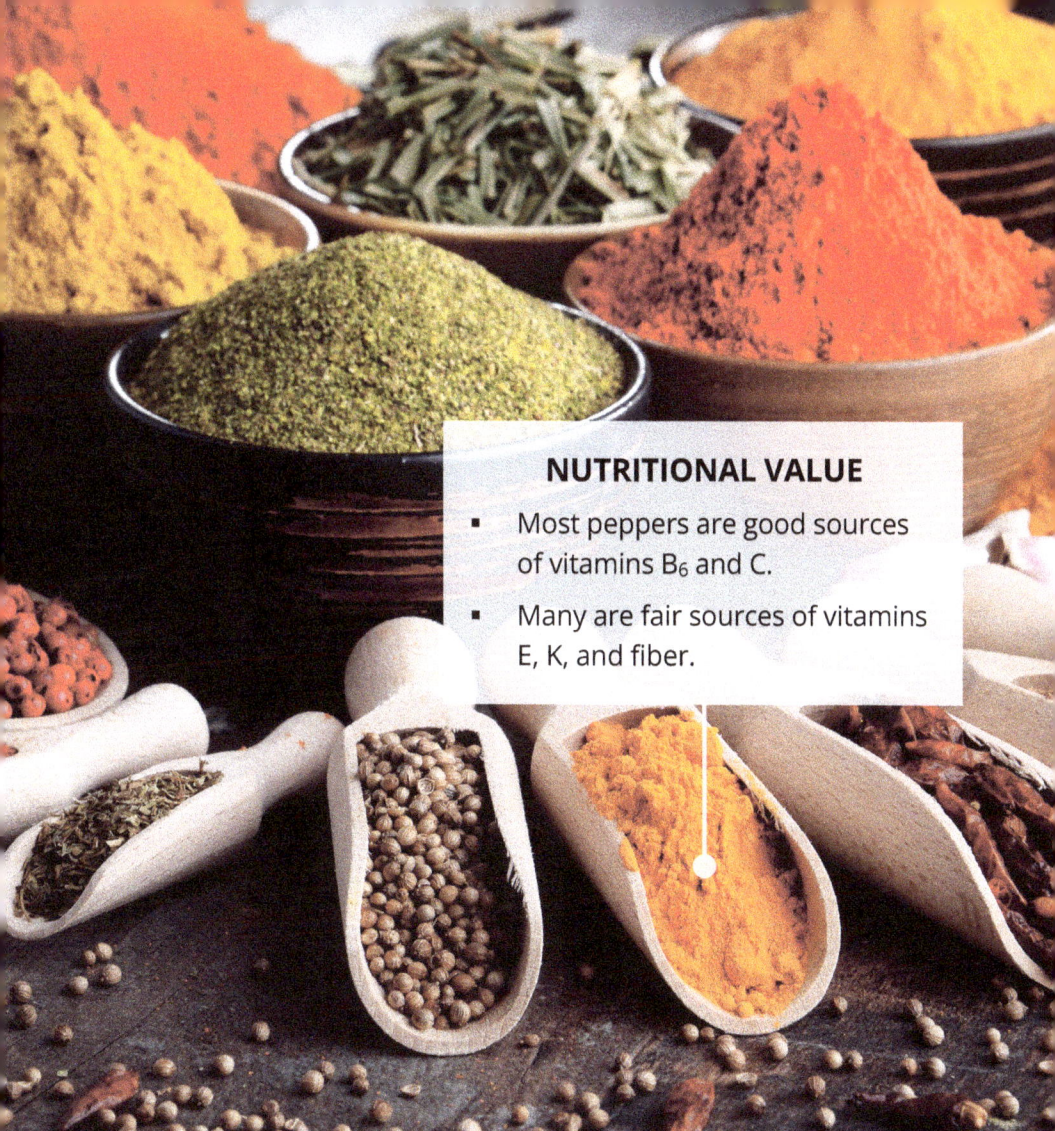

NUTRITIONAL VALUE
- Most peppers are good sources of vitamins B_6 and C.
- Many are fair sources of vitamins E, K, and fiber.

25 Peppers & Spices

Common Avoidance *Responses*

- Gas
- Bloating
- Abdominal discomfort
- Lip or tongue swelling
- Hives or other skin reactions

Food Clue *Category*

- Poor liver function
- Poor protein digestion

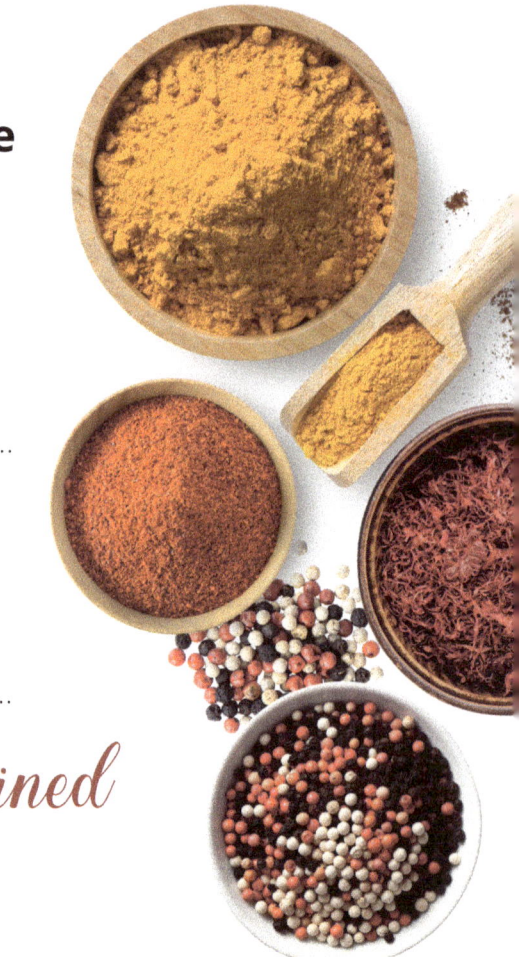

Food Clue *Explained*

One cause of pepper and spice avoidance is related to the poor breakdown of capsaicin by the liver. Capsaicin is the natural chemical in peppers and spices that produces the hot and burning sensation and is a nitrogen-based compound. Nitrogen breakdown occurs in the liver by the uric cycle, so if that cycle becomes dysfunctional due to infection, inflammation, etc., it could result in a reduced ability to manage nitrogen and sensitivity or avoidance of nitrogen-based compounds.

HEALTH CONCERNS

- Liver or gallbladder dysfunction
- Difficulty losing weight
- Chronic constipation
- Digestive conditions including irritable bowel syndrome, Crohn's disease, celiac disease

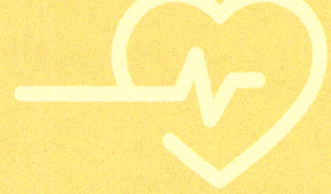

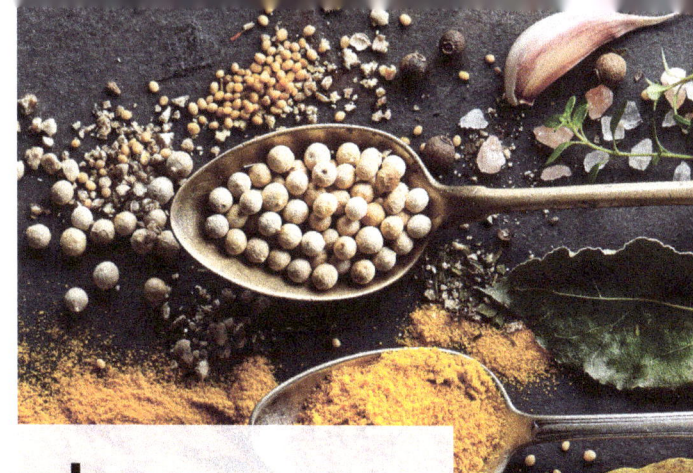

Additional
Information

Sensitivity and avoidance of chili peppers can also be due to difficulty with protein breakdown, as many have specific plant protein compounds in them associated with sensitivity and allergic reactions (e.g., profilin protein).

Lastly, peppers are also members of the nightshade food category. Nightshade foods contain significant amounts of nitrogen, which can result in symptoms if the uric cycle in the liver is dysfunctional. Poor uric cycle performance can create poor breakdown and elimination of excess nitrogen, causing a backup of nitrogen in the liver.

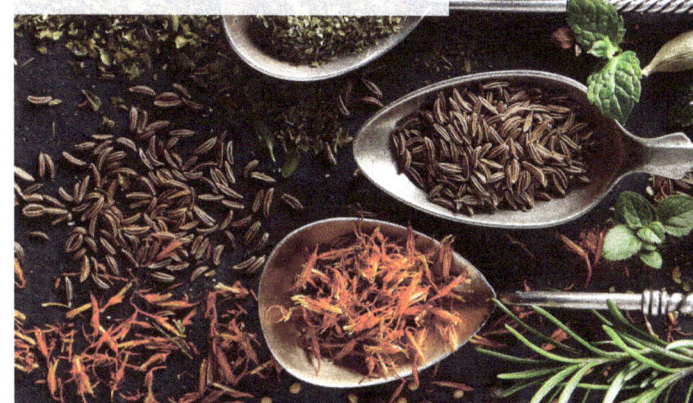

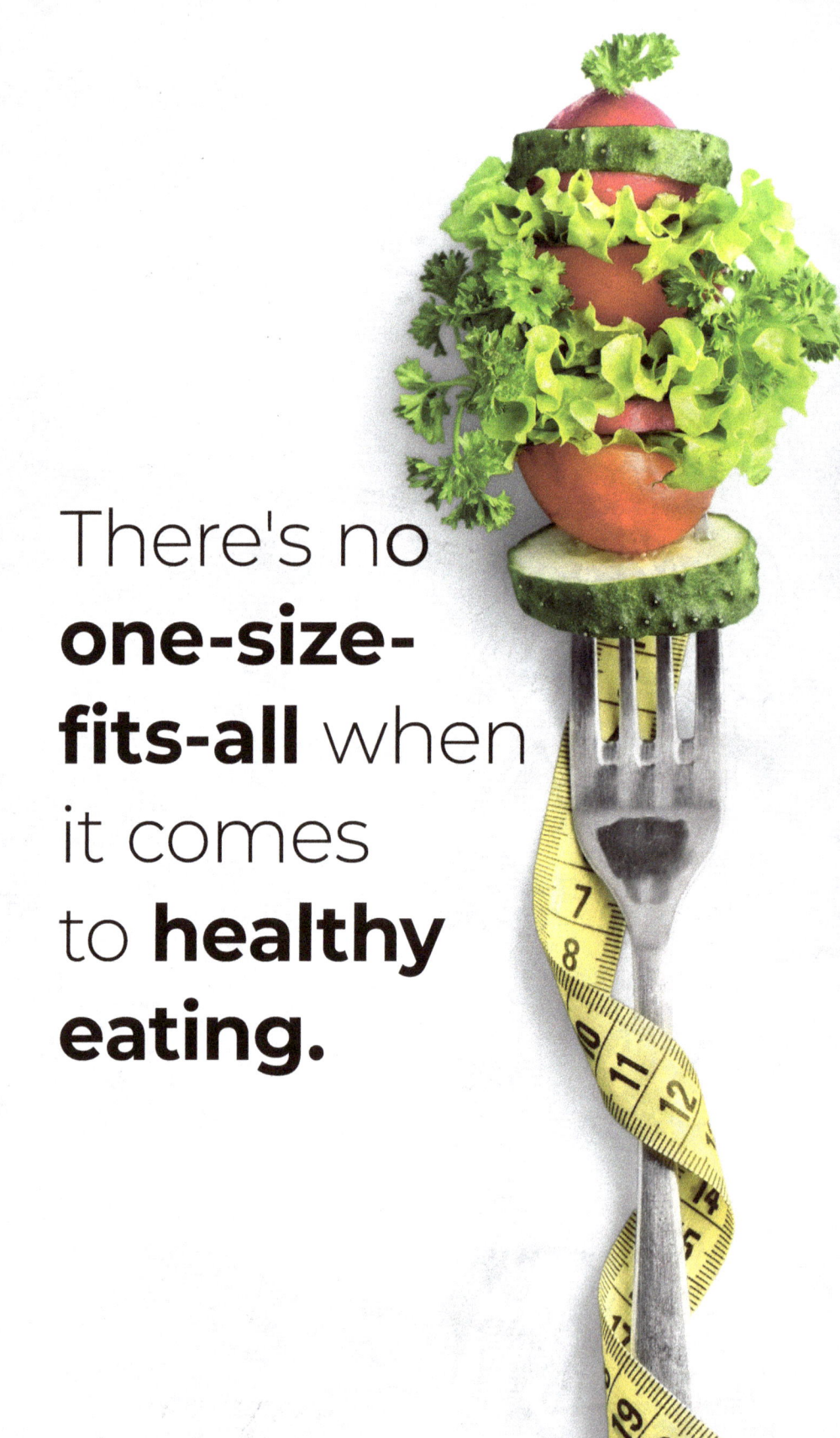

There's no **one-size-fits-all** when it comes to **healthy eating.**

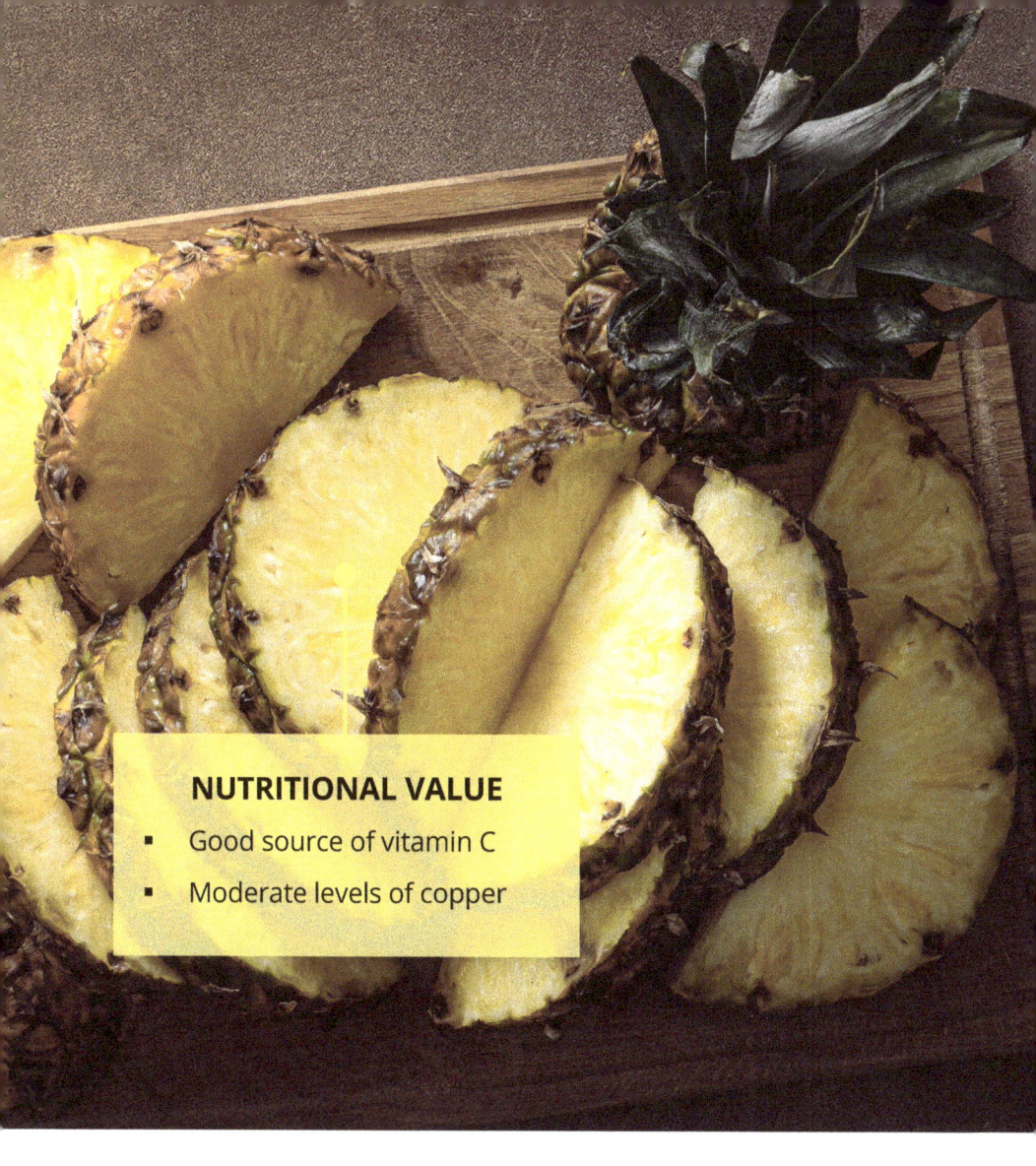

NUTRITIONAL VALUE
- Good source of vitamin C
- Moderate levels of copper

26 Pineapple

Common Avoidance *Responses*

- Abdominal discomfort
- Lip or tongue swelling
- Hives or other skin reactions

Food Clue *Category*

- Poor protein digestion
- Metal toxicity

HEALTH CONCERNS

- Liver or gallbladder dysfunction
- Difficulty losing weight
- Chronic constipation
- Digestive conditions including irritable bowel syndrome, Crohn's disease, celiac disease

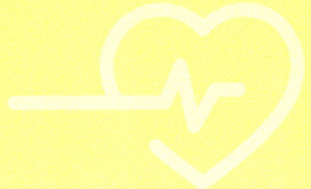

Food Clue *Explained*

Sensitivity to and avoidance of pineapple is due to difficulty with protein breakdown, as it has specific plant proteins in it that are associated with sensitivity and allergic reactions (e.g., profilin protein).

Additional *Information*

There can also be reactions in those with high metal loads in their systems, due to its moderate levels of copper.

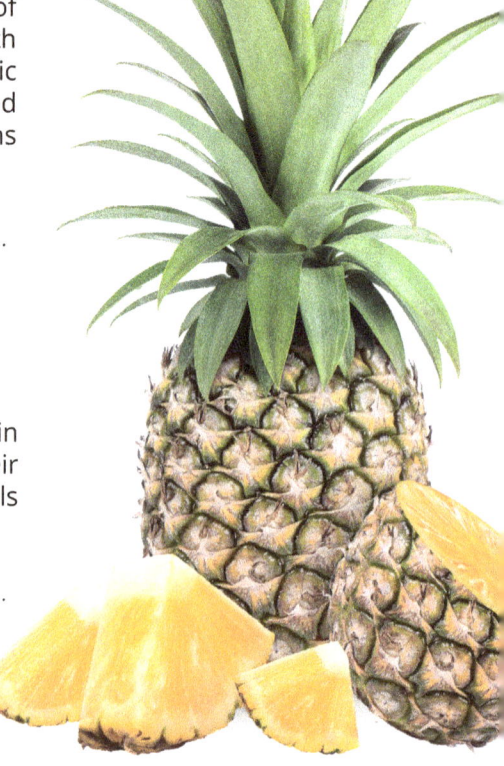

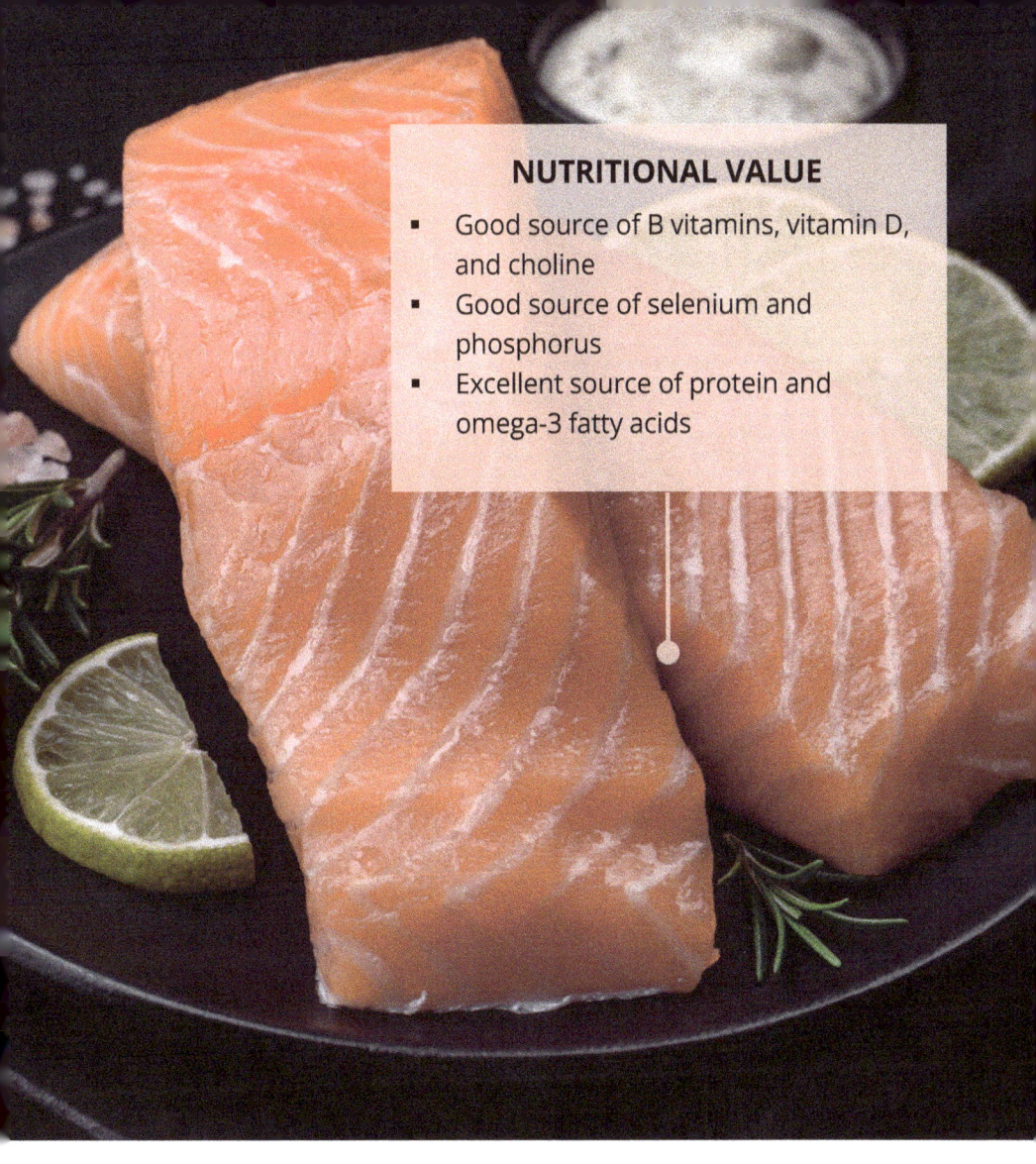

NUTRITIONAL VALUE

- Good source of B vitamins, vitamin D, and choline
- Good source of selenium and phosphorus
- Excellent source of protein and omega-3 fatty acids

27 Salmon & Other Fish

Common Avoidance *Responses*

- Difficulty chewing (Many will say it's a texture thing)
- General avoidance

Food Clue *Category*

- Poor protein digestion

HEALTH CONCERNS

- Small intestinal bacterial overgrowth (SIBO)
- Digestive conditions including irritable bowel syndrome, Crohn's disease, celiac disease
- Emotional and mental health imbalances including anxiety, depression, autism, attention deficit disorder, attention deficit hyperactivity disorder

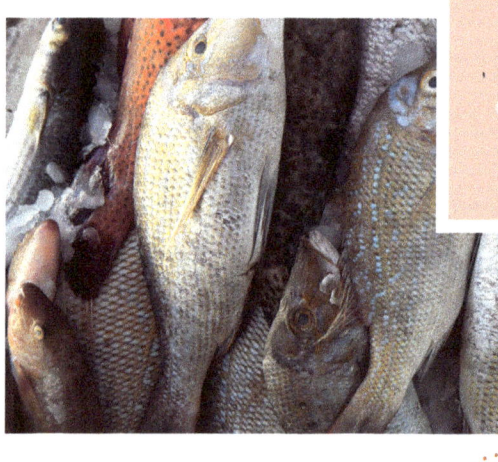

Food Clue *Explained*

Similar to other protein-based ingredients like steak, avoidance of salmon suggests difficulty with protein digestion, including difficulty with acid breakdown, acid elimination, or an overload of acid. Salmon has almost twice the amount of protein as steak in each serving.

Allergy *Stats*

- Fish allergies are considered a top fourteen allergen by the National Institute of Health.
- Self-reports of fish allergies are stated at 0.4%, whereas other reports state fish allergies totaling 1% of the US population

Additional
Information

Reaction and avoidance commonly occur due to infections, often concentrated in the stomach and small intestine, which disrupt digestion.

Other causes of reactions to fish include elevated metal loads in the body, as fish can contain higher levels of mercury than other meats, so avoidance of additional metals in the system may occur. Other toxins and microorganism infections from ocean pollution and other sources can contribute to avoidance reactions to fish.

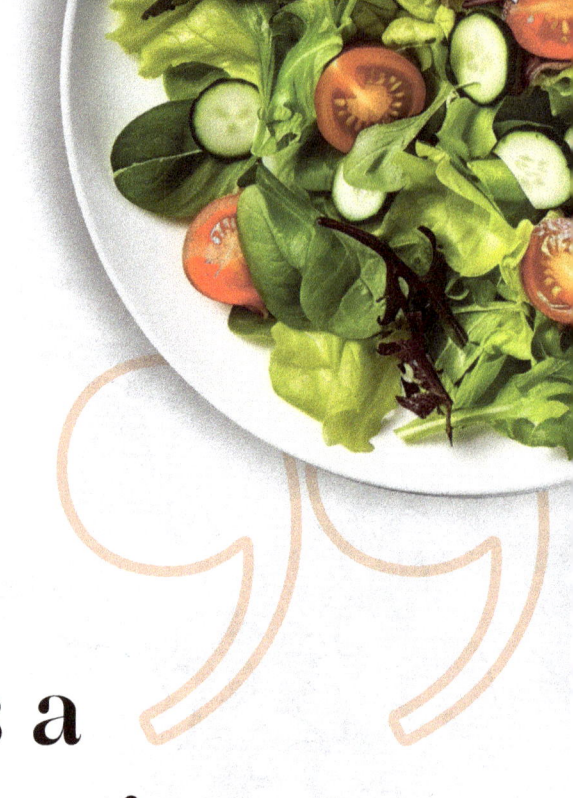

Food is a conversation between you and your body. What are saying to yourself?

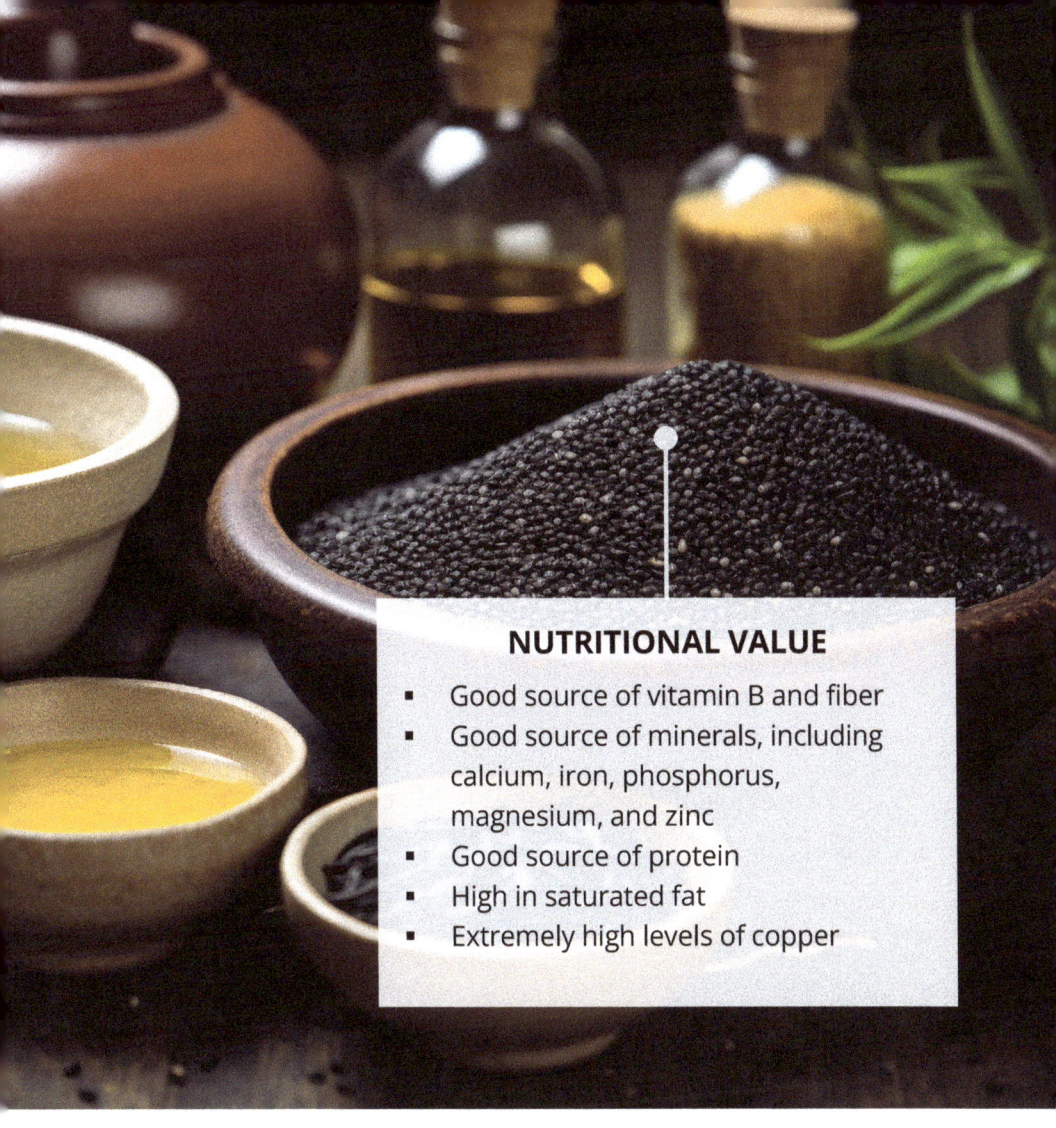

NUTRITIONAL VALUE

- Good source of vitamin B and fiber
- Good source of minerals, including calcium, iron, phosphorus, magnesium, and zinc
- Good source of protein
- High in saturated fat
- Extremely high levels of copper

28 Sesame

Common Avoidance *Responses*

- Lip or tongue swelling
- Itchy skin
- Gas, bloating, or nausea
- Anaphylactic responses in extreme cases

Food Clue *Category*

- Fatty acid imbalance
- Poor protein digestion
- Poor acid management

HEALTH CONCERNS

- Small intestinal bacterial overgrowth (SIBO)
- Estrogen imbalance
- Menstrual cycle dysfunction or conditions including heavy bleeding, missed cycles, endometriosis, and polycystic ovary syndrome (PCOS)
- Digestive conditions including irritable bowel syndrome, Crohn's disease, celiac disease
- Emotional and mental health imbalances including anxiety, depression, autism, attention deficit disorder, attention deficit hyperactivity disorder

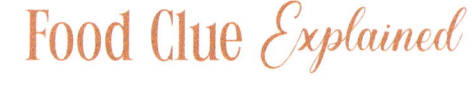

Similar to tree nuts and peanuts, reactions to sesame, particularly sesame oil, can indicate an imbalance in omega-6 and omega-3 fatty acids. In general, the body prefers a ratio of omega-6 to omega-3 levels closer to 3:1, and most often there's an excess of omega-6 fatty acid relative to omega-3 levels when avoidance reactions occur. Sesame oil has an omega ratio close to 130:1.

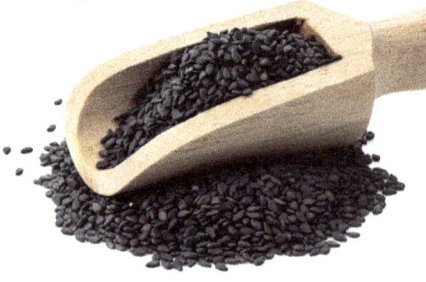

A common reason for fatty acid imbalance can be an unhealthy diet, particularly one that includes high levels of processed foods, which often have much higher levels of omega-6 than omega-3 fatty acids. Research has shown that diets high in processed foods, which are common in the United States, can have omega-6 to omega-3 ratios up to five times the normal ratio.

Diets high in omega-6 fatty acids can increase inflammatory cell performance and break down the intestinal lining, also known as "leaky gut." This can allow toxins and germs to escape through the thin lining into the bloodstream, travel to other areas of the body and set the stage for organ dysfunction and system illness or disease.

Allergy *Stats*

- Effective January 2023, sesame is considered a top allergen by the National Institute of Health
- Recent reports state that about 0.2% of the US population is allergic to sesame

Additional *Information*

Similar to peanuts, sesame is high in fat and protein, it also means that they are considerably acidic, as fats breakdown to fatty acids and proteins break down to amino acids. Therefore it's likely that sesame allergies could also be an indicator of poor acid management in the body.

Poor acid management often results in poor acid elimination. Unlike carbs, sugars, and some vitamins and minerals, the human body has little to no capacity to store excess acids and many acidic compounds are supposed to be used and the excess eliminated. If excess acids aren't properly eliminated the backup can cause body performance issues but more importantly the body will protect itself by utilizing avoidance or protective mechanisms to prevent you from ingesting more acids that it can't process likely resulting in the allergic response.

It's likely that anaphylaxis is a severe response to an extremely significant acid management issue; a key cell that recognizes problematic substances in the body (IgE) may be excessively released in an excessive attempt to prevent the introduction of more acid based substances into the body.

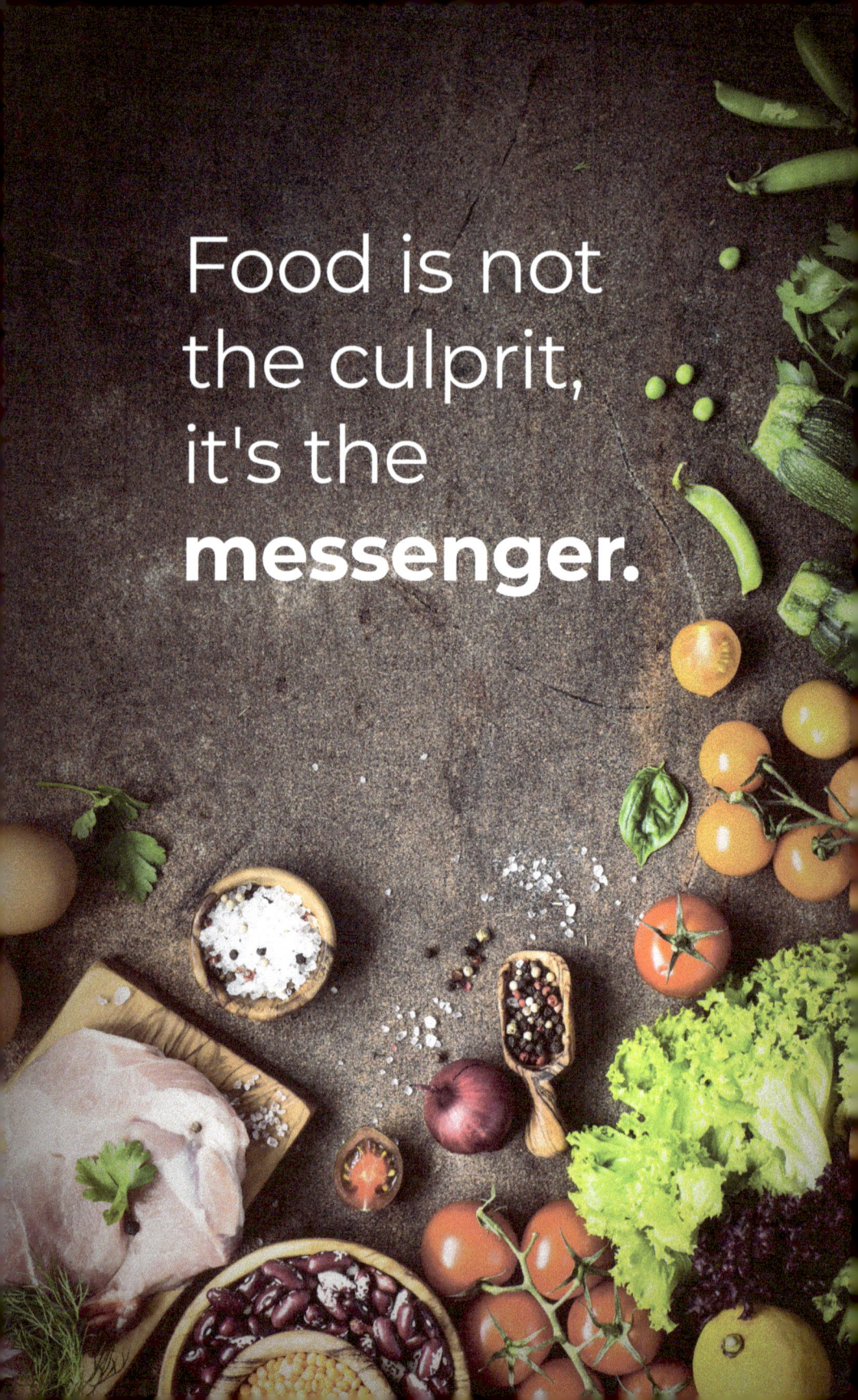

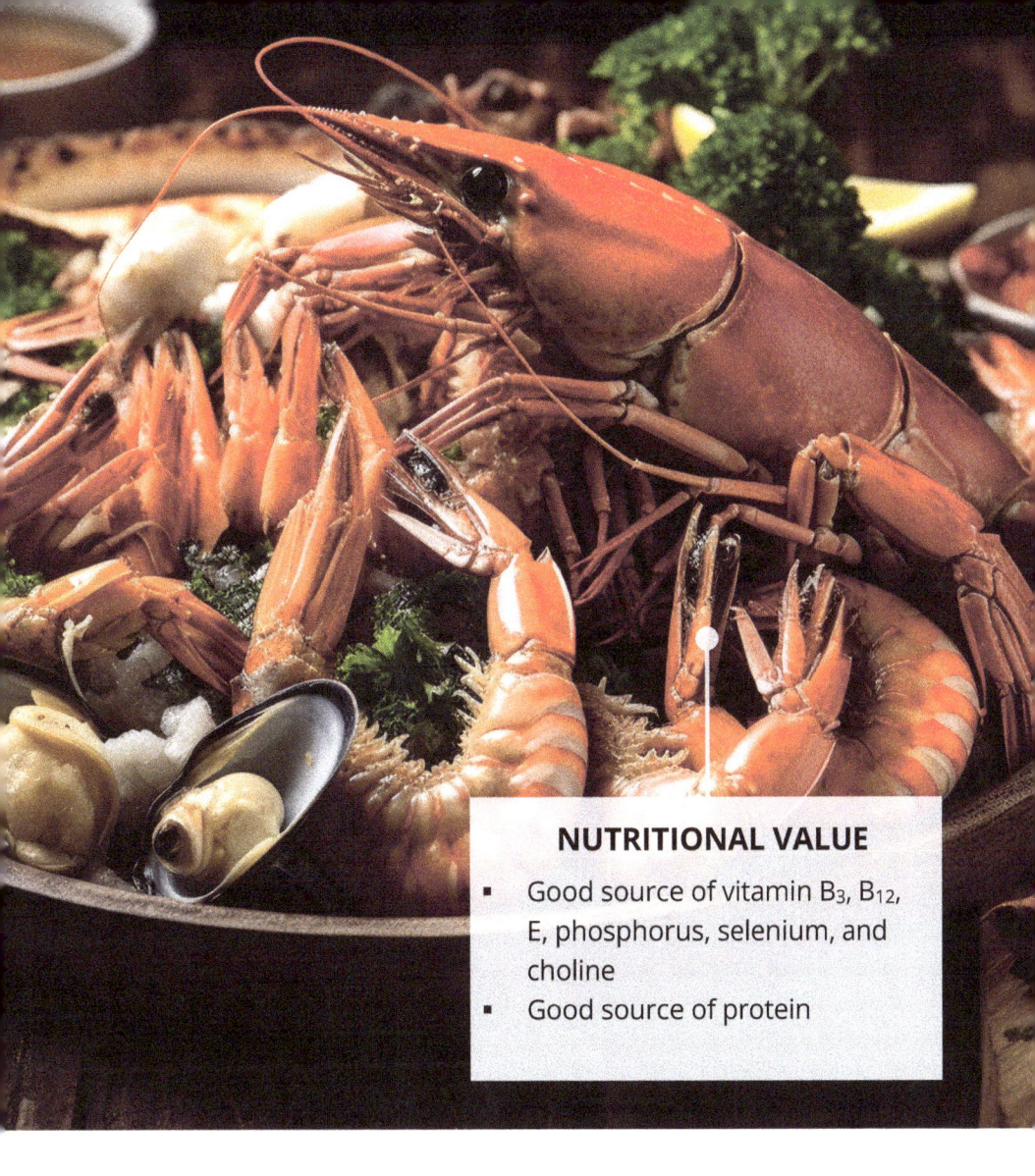

NUTRITIONAL VALUE
- Good source of vitamin B_3, B_{12}, E, phosphorus, selenium, and choline
- Good source of protein

29 Shrimp & Other Shellfish

Common Avoidance *Responses*

- Lip or tongue swelling
- Itchy skin
- Gas, bloating, or nausea
- Anaphylactic responses in extreme cases

Food Clue *Category*

- Metal toxicity
- Poor protein digestion

Allergy *Stats*

- Crustacean fish are considered a top allergen by the National Institute of Health.
- The National Library of Medicine states about 14% of individuals have a shellfish allergy.
- Accurate reports can be clouded by reactions to other toxins and substances in shellfish rather than the fish itself.

Food Clue *Explained*

Many fish allergies, including those to shrimp and other shellfish, are due to difficulty digesting certain proteins that are more common to fish (e.g., parvalbumin, tropomyosin, enolases, aldolases, collagen, and gelatin).

HEALTH CONCERNS

- Liver or gallbladder dysfunction
- Digestive conditions including irritable bowel syndrome, Crohn's disease, celiac disease

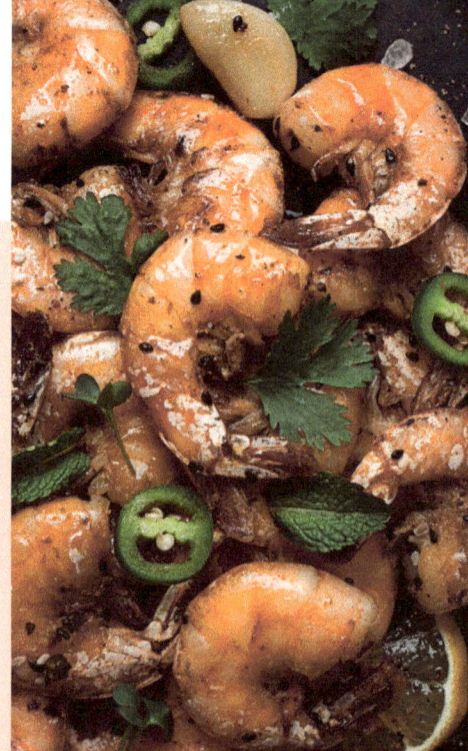

Additional
Information

Other causes of reactions to shellfish include elevated metal loads in the body, as shellfish can contain higher levels of mercury than other meats, so avoidance of additional metals in the system may occur.

Shrimp are also high in fat and cholesterol, so poor liver function can also contribute to avoidance responses of fish and shellfish. Finally, other toxins and microorganism infections from ocean pollution and other sources can contribute to avoidance reactions to shellfish.

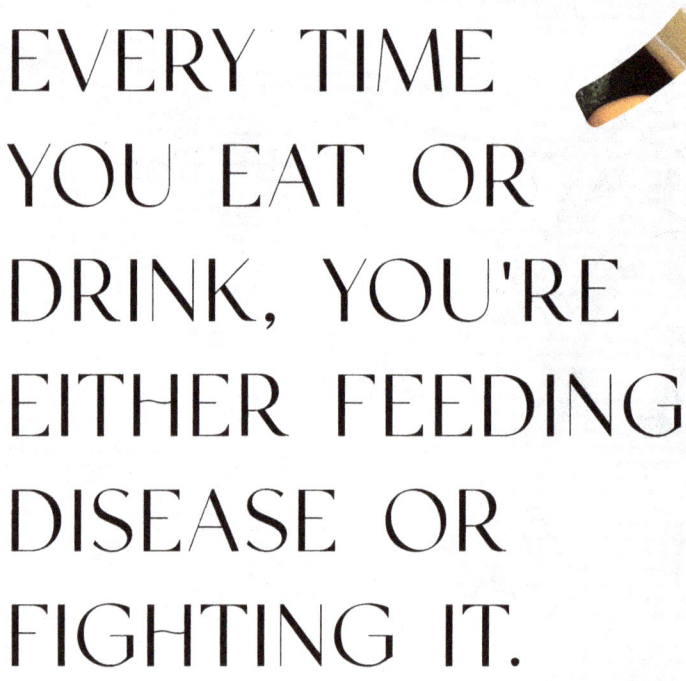

EVERY TIME YOU EAT OR DRINK, YOU'RE EITHER FEEDING DISEASE OR FIGHTING IT.

- HEATHER MORGAN

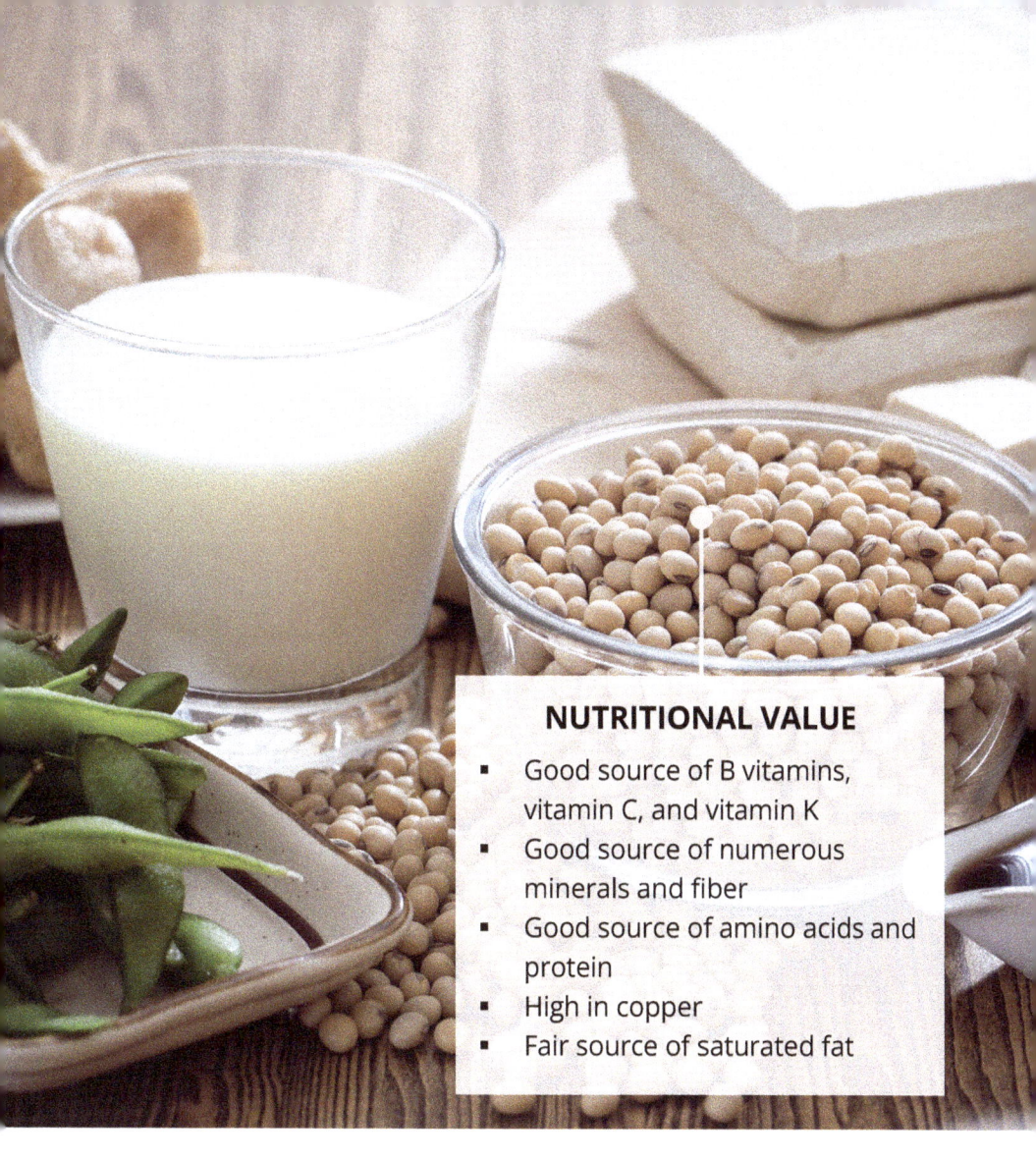

NUTRITIONAL VALUE

- Good source of B vitamins, vitamin C, and vitamin K
- Good source of numerous minerals and fiber
- Good source of amino acids and protein
- High in copper
- Fair source of saturated fat

30 Soy

Common Avoidance *Responses*

- Gas
- Bloating
- Indigestion
- Constipation
- Abdominal pain
- Nausea

Food Clue *Category*

- Poor protein digestion

Allergy *Stats*

- Soy bean is considered a top allergen by the National Institute of Health
- Most statistics refer to children, reporting anywhere from 0.5%–1.1% occurrence in children, and even less in adults

Food Clue *Explained*

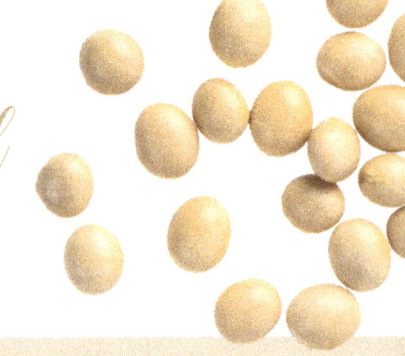

Intolerance to soy is often a sign of difficulty with digesting common plant proteins like profilin, but also includes those specific to beans that come in pods. Reactions to certain beans are often related to the complexity of the protein compounds in the bean, so you can have reactions to some beans but not to others.

HEALTH CONCERNS

- Small intestinal bacterial overgrowth (SIBO)
- Digestive conditions including irritable bowel syndrome, Crohn's disease, celiac disease
- Emotional and mental health imbalances including anxiety, depression, autism, attention deficit disorder, attention deficit hyperactivity disorder

Additional *Information*

Soybean oil has an omega-6 to omega-3 ratio of around 7:1, so there can also be signs of dysbiosis (unbalanced digestive bacterial levels in the gut) due to elevated bacterial levels associated with elevated omega-6 levels in the body.

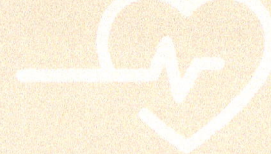

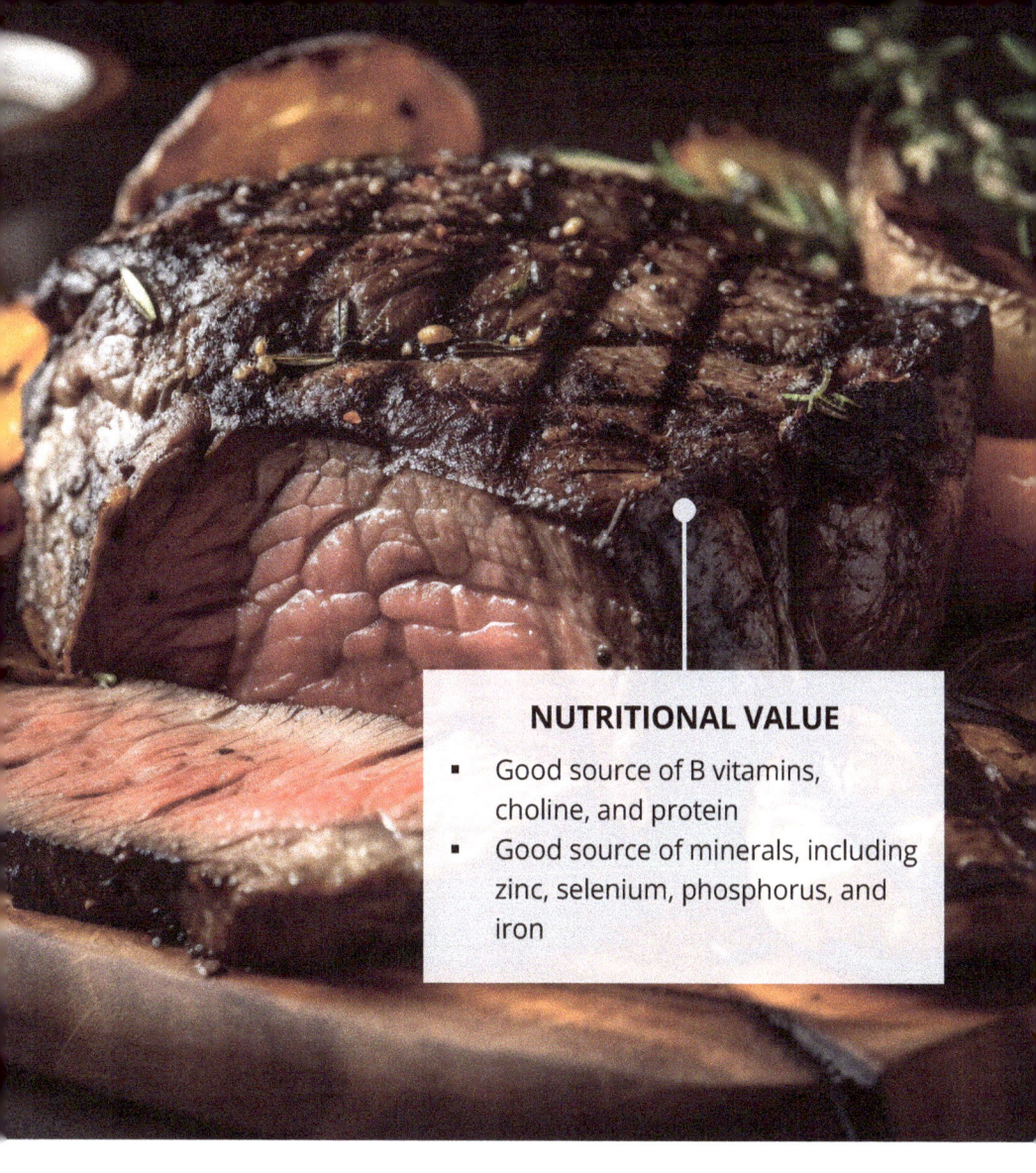

NUTRITIONAL VALUE

- Good source of B vitamins, choline, and protein
- Good source of minerals, including zinc, selenium, phosphorus, and iron

31 Steak

Common Avoidance *Responses*

- Difficulty chewing (Many will say it's a texture thing.)
- Gas
- Bloating
- Abdominal discomfort

Food Clue *Category*

- Poor protein digestion

HEALTH CONCERNS

- Small intestinal bacterial overgrowth (SIBO)
- Digestive conditions including irritable bowel syndrome, Crohn's disease, celiac disease
- Emotional and mental health imbalances including anxiety, depression, autism, attention deficit disorder, attention deficit hyperactivity disorder

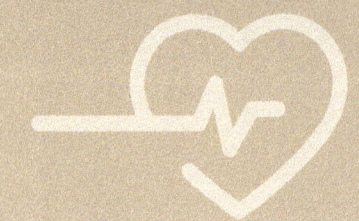

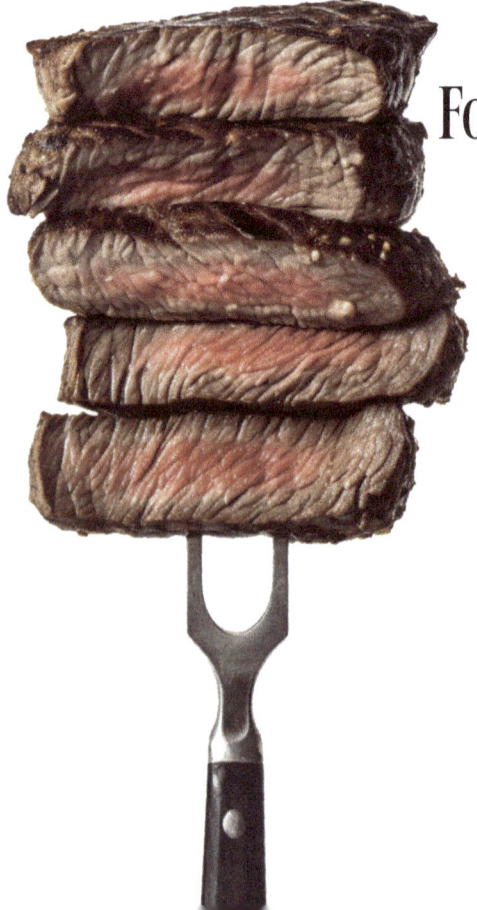

Food Clue *Explained*

Avoidance of steak suggests difficulty with protein digestion. Reactions can also suggest difficulty with acid breakdown or elimination, or indicate an overload of acid, resulting in an avoidance reaction against eating steak since the building blocks of proteins are amino acids.

Steak avoidance can also be related to elevated histamine levels in the body because proteins contain histidine, which is the precursor to histamine, the immune response that produces itching, rashes, and hives in response to a germ or other irritant.

FOOD CLUES 113

Additional
Information

Steak reactions and avoidance commonly occur due to infections, often concentrated in the stomach and small intestine, which disrupt digestion. Steak reactions could also indicate exposure to acidic chemicals, raising the overall acidity of the body, resulting in avoidance of or reactions to anything acidic.

Nausea or headache within the first few bites or after catching a whiff of steak are also common dislike symptoms. Some people get symptoms even with the thought of eating steak. Responses like these are more of a nervous system response, alerting you against putting something in your body that your body knows is harmful in some way.

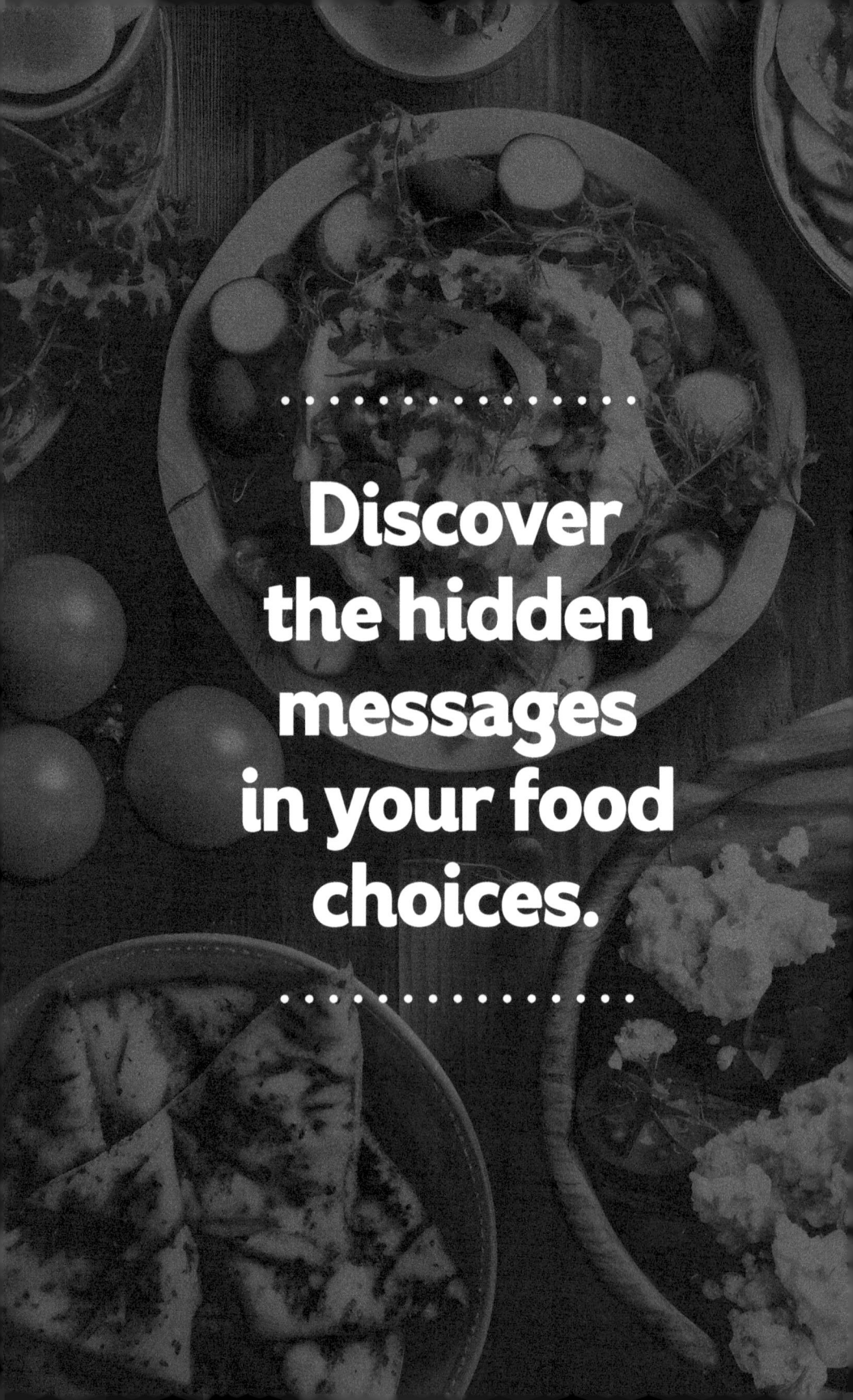

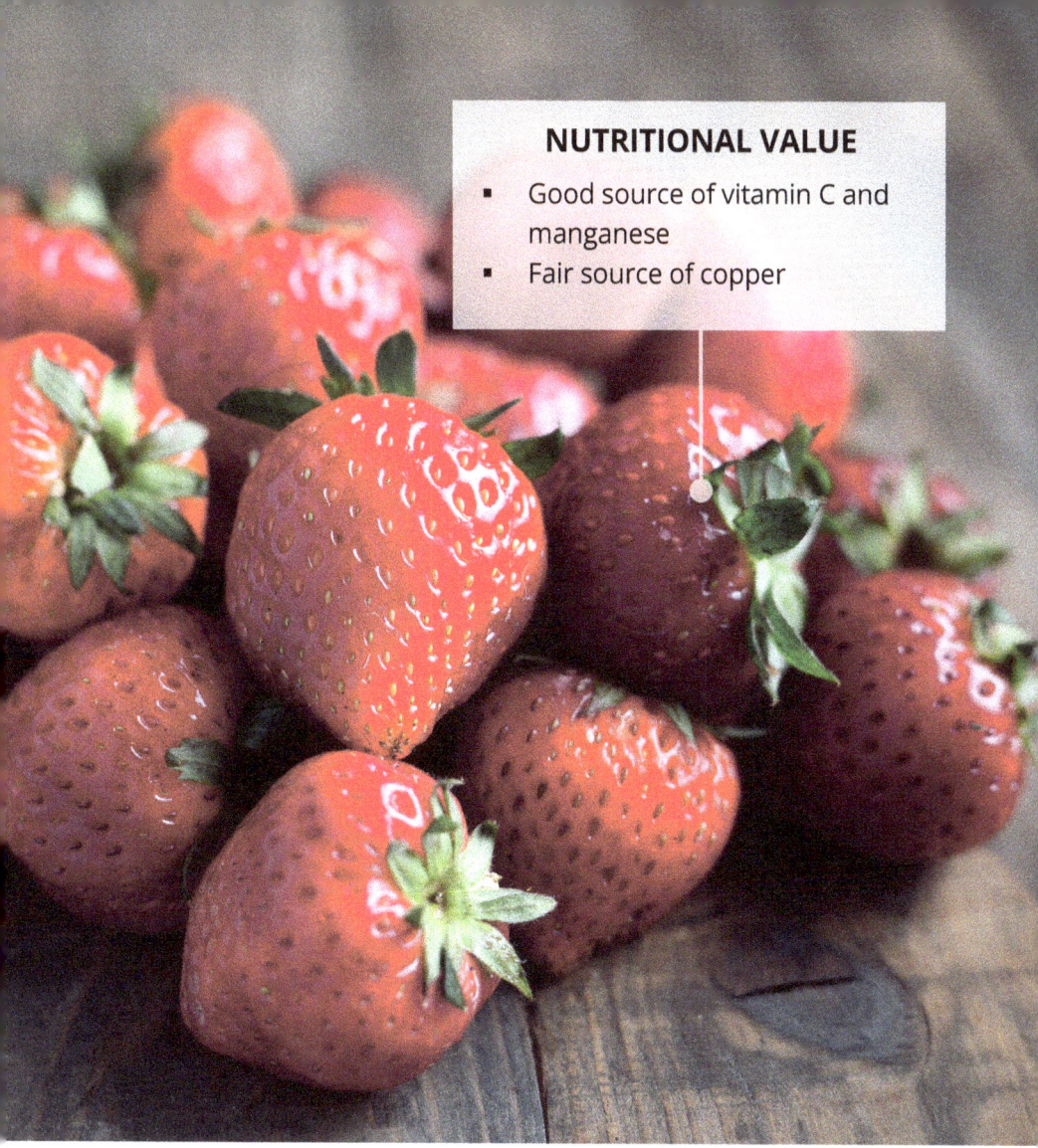

NUTRITIONAL VALUE
- Good source of vitamin C and manganese
- Fair source of copper

32 Strawberries

Common Avoidance *Responses*

- Gas
- Bloating
- Abdominal discomfort
- Lip or tongue swelling
- Hives or other skin reactions

Food Clue *Category*

- Unbalanced immune system

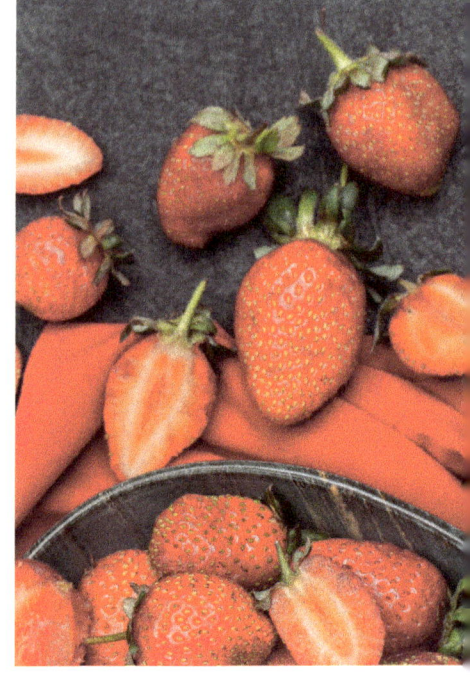

Food Clue *Explained*

A common cause of strawberry reactions is due to elevated histamine levels in the body. Histamines stimulate stomach acid secretion, help reduce inflammation, dilate blood vessels, support muscle contractions in the intestines and lungs, and influence heart rate. If any of the other organs or systems driving those functions become impaired, histamine levels may be boosted as compensation to keep those functions going.

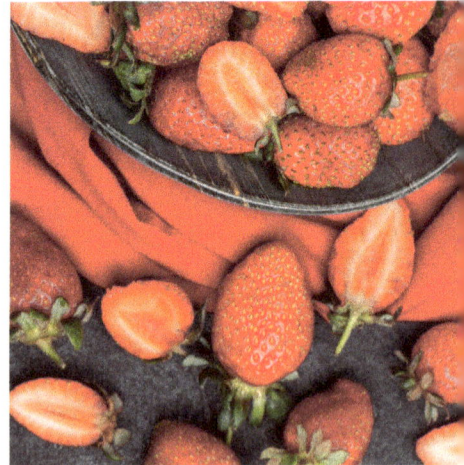

HEALTH CONCERNS

- Autoimmune conditions
- Liver or gallbladder dysfunction
- Mast cell activation syndrome

Additional
Information

The biggest driver of elevated histamine levels and strawberry avoidance is infection. Whether there are multiple infections collecting over time or one is acquired as another resolves, persistent issues resolving infection is a primary cause of elevated histamines in the body.

Avoidance of strawberries can also be related to infection through bug contamination, making thorough washing of strawberries crucial before consumption. Lastly, strawberries also contain profilin, a common plant protein known to create difficulty with digestion, resulting in sensitivity and avoidance.

"It's never too late or never too early to work towards being the healthiest you"

~ Anonymous

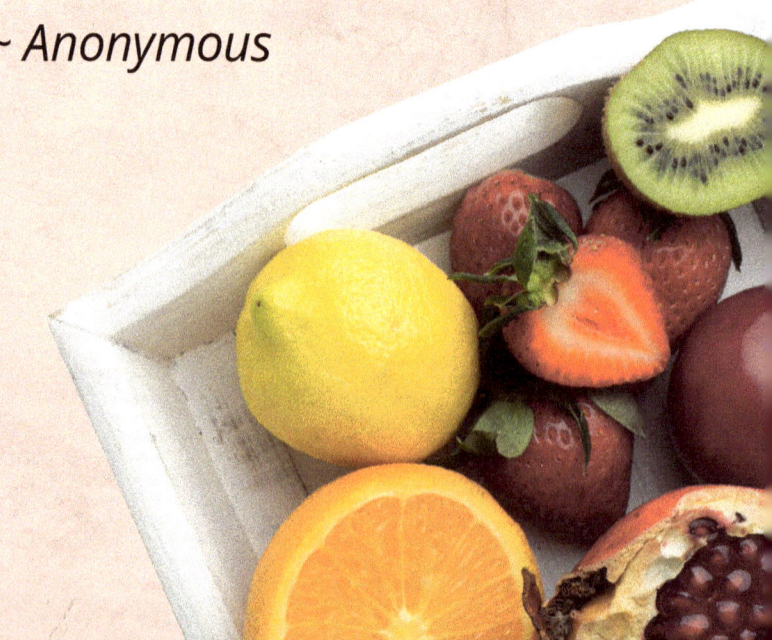

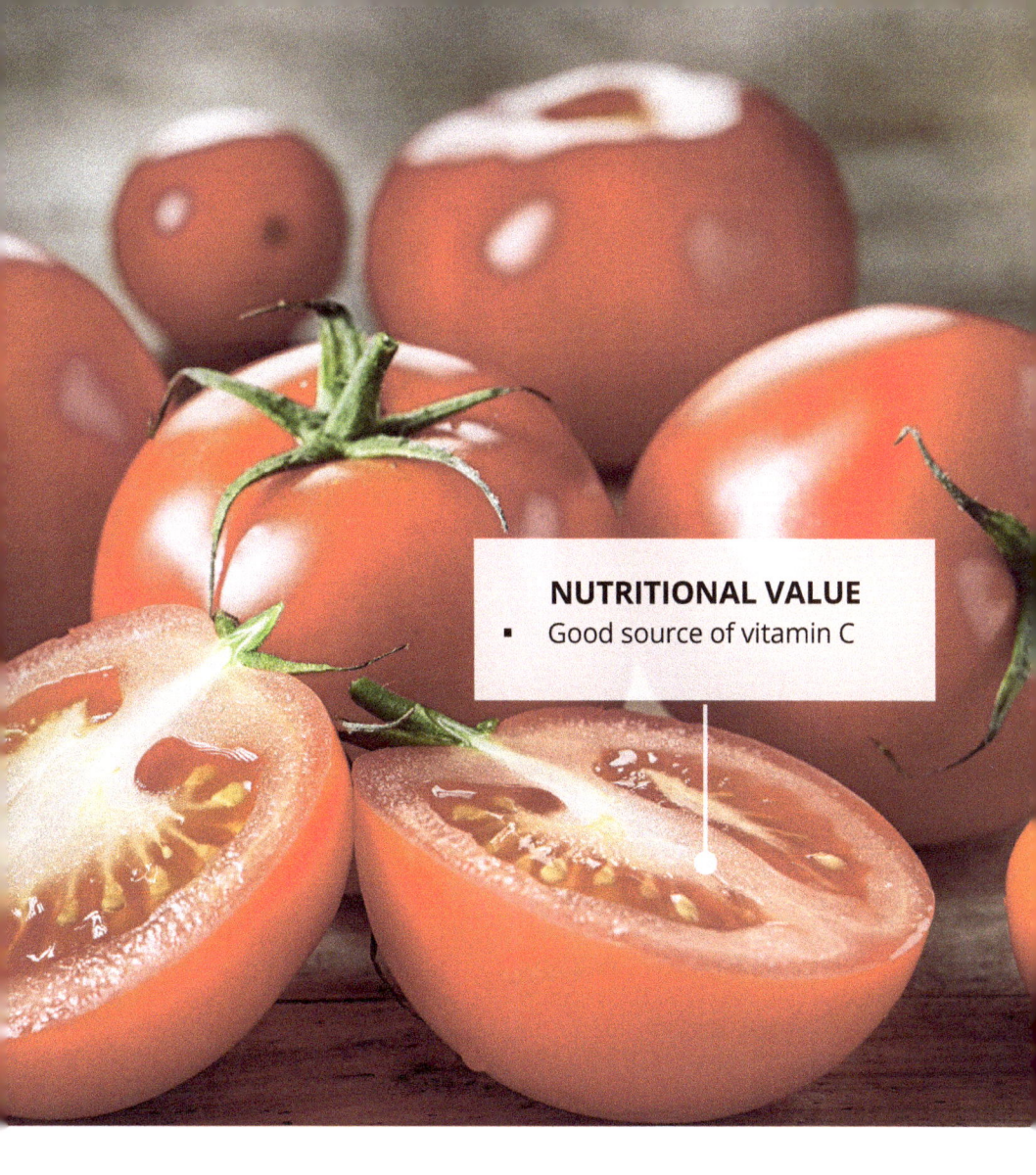

NUTRITIONAL VALUE
- Good source of vitamin C

33 Tomatoes

Common Avoidance *Responses*

- General avoidance

Food Clue *Category*

- Poor protein digestion
- Poor liver function
- Poor acid management

Food Clue *Explained*

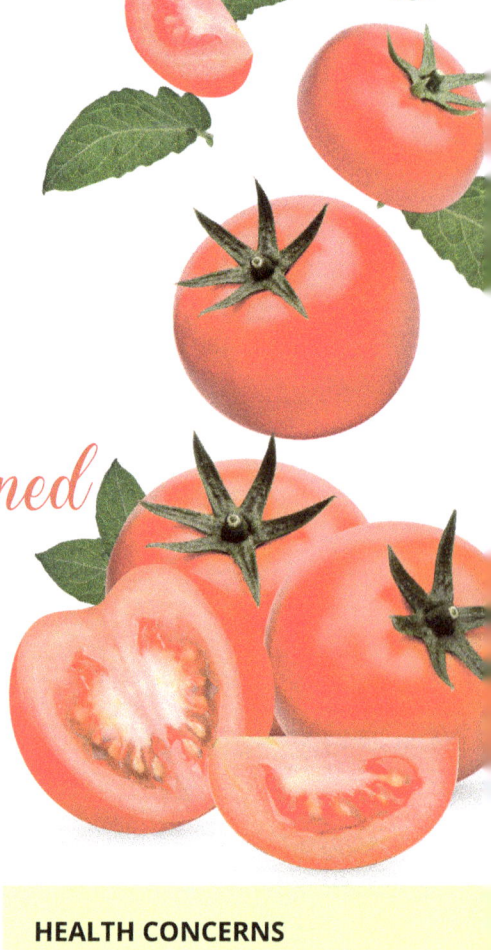

While traditional allergies are low across the world, many people avoid tomatoes, likely due to their acidic content. Tomatoes have a pH averaging 4.5, so people who avoid them may do so due to thin or inflamed stomach or intestinal lining, which becomes more irritated when acids come into contact with it. An impaired stomach lining may also cause a decreased release of digestive juices, which are typically acidic in nature, resulting in difficulty with digestion.

Avoidance of tomatoes can also be related to elevated histamine levels in the body, signaling that immune performance may be impaired.

HEALTH CONCERNS

- Liver or gallbladder dysfunction
- Gastrointestinal ulcers
- Gastroesophageal reflux disease (GERD)

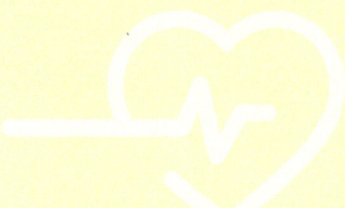

FOOD CLUES

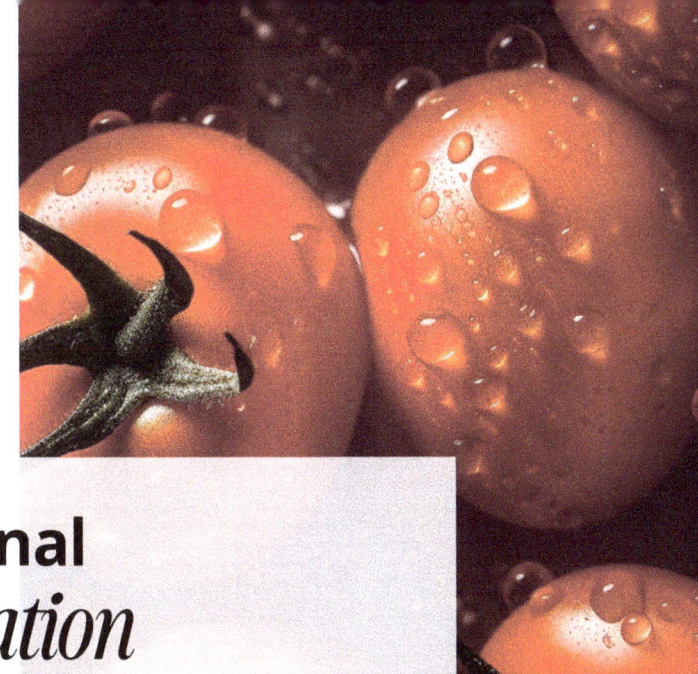

Additional
Information

Tomatoes contain profilin, a common plant protein known to create difficulty with digestion, resulting in sensitivity and avoidance. Lastly, tomatoes are also members of the nightshade food category. Nightshade foods contain significant amounts of nitrogen, which can result in symptoms if the uric cycle in the liver is dysfunctional. Poor uric cycle performance can create poor breakdown and elimination of excess nitrogen, causing a backup of nitrogen in the liver.

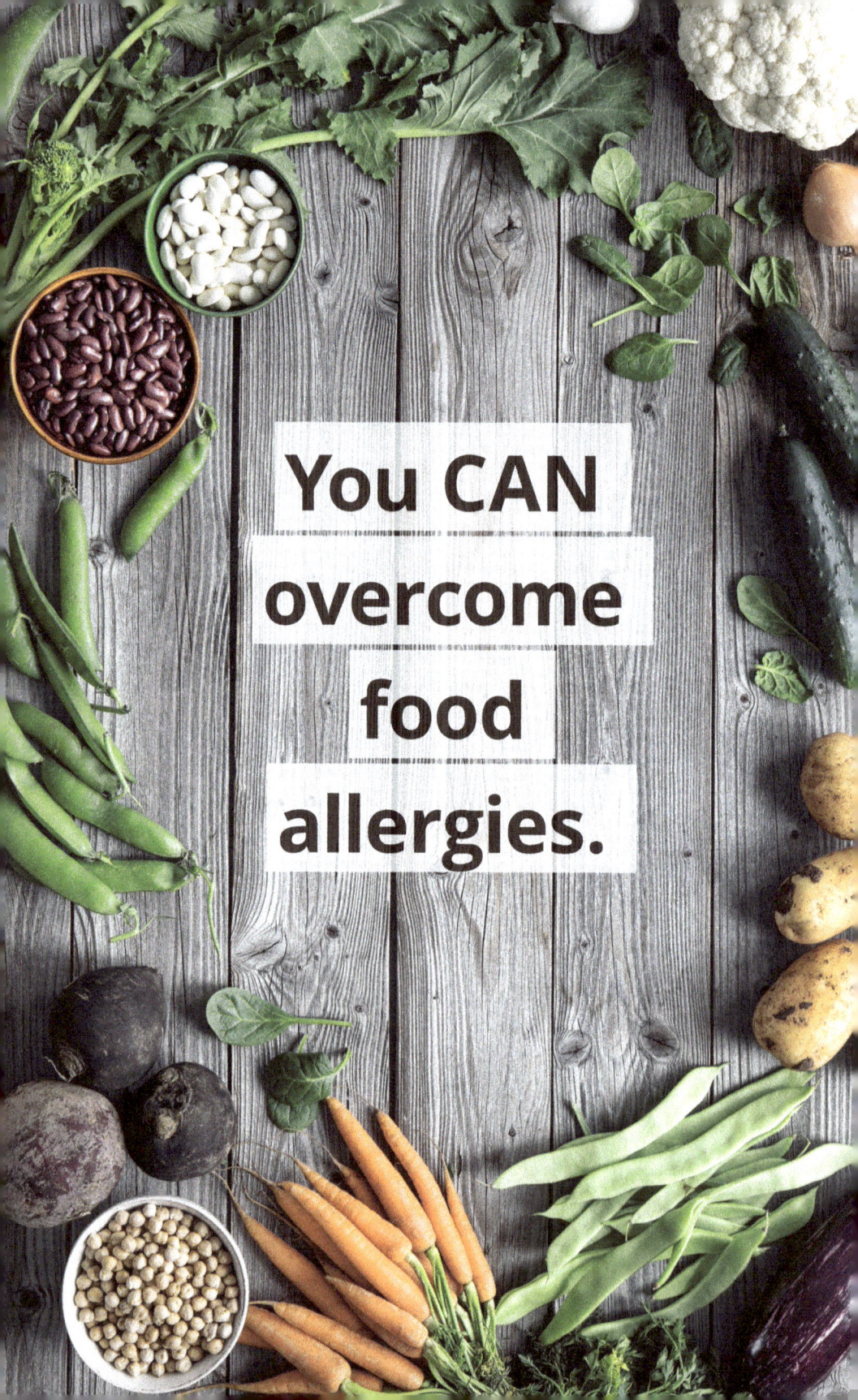

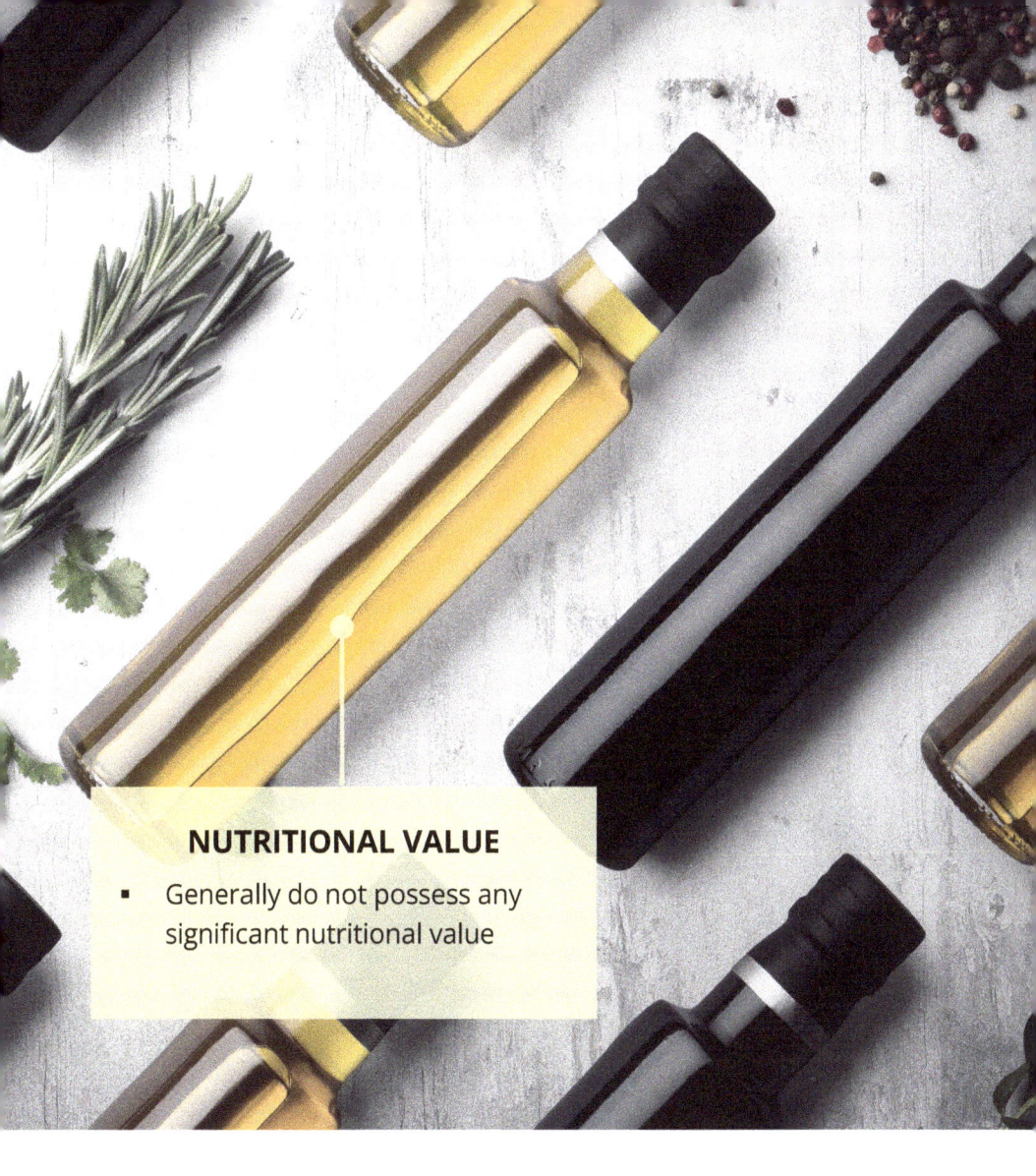

NUTRITIONAL VALUE
- Generally do not possess any significant nutritional value

34 Vinegar

Common Avoidance *Responses*

- General avoidance

Food Clue *Category*

- Poor general digestion
- Poor acid management

HEALTH CONCERNS

- Gastrointestinal ulcers
- Gastroesophageal reflux disease (GERD)

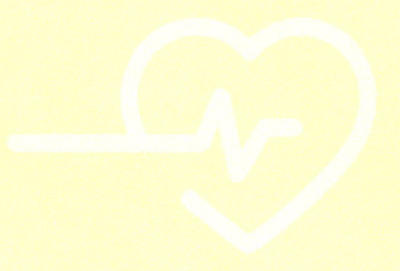

Food Clue *Explained*

Similar to those who avoid lemons, many people avoid vinegar and foods made with vinegar due to their acidic content. Vinegar has a pH averaging 2.5, so just like with lemons, people who avoid vinegar may do so due to thin or inflamed stomach or intestinal lining, which becomes more irritated when acids come into contact with it. Low stomach lining may also cause a decreased release of bile and other digestive juices, which are typically acidic in nature, resulting in difficulty with the digestion of fats and other substances.

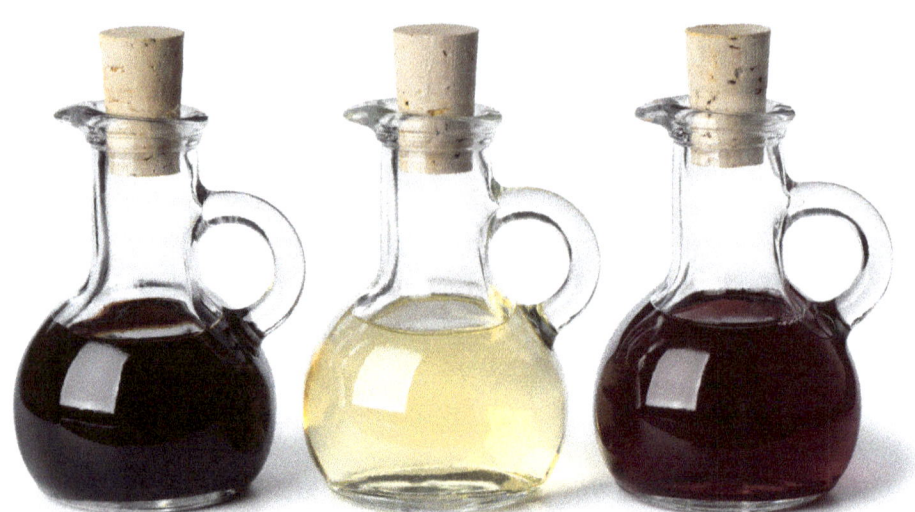

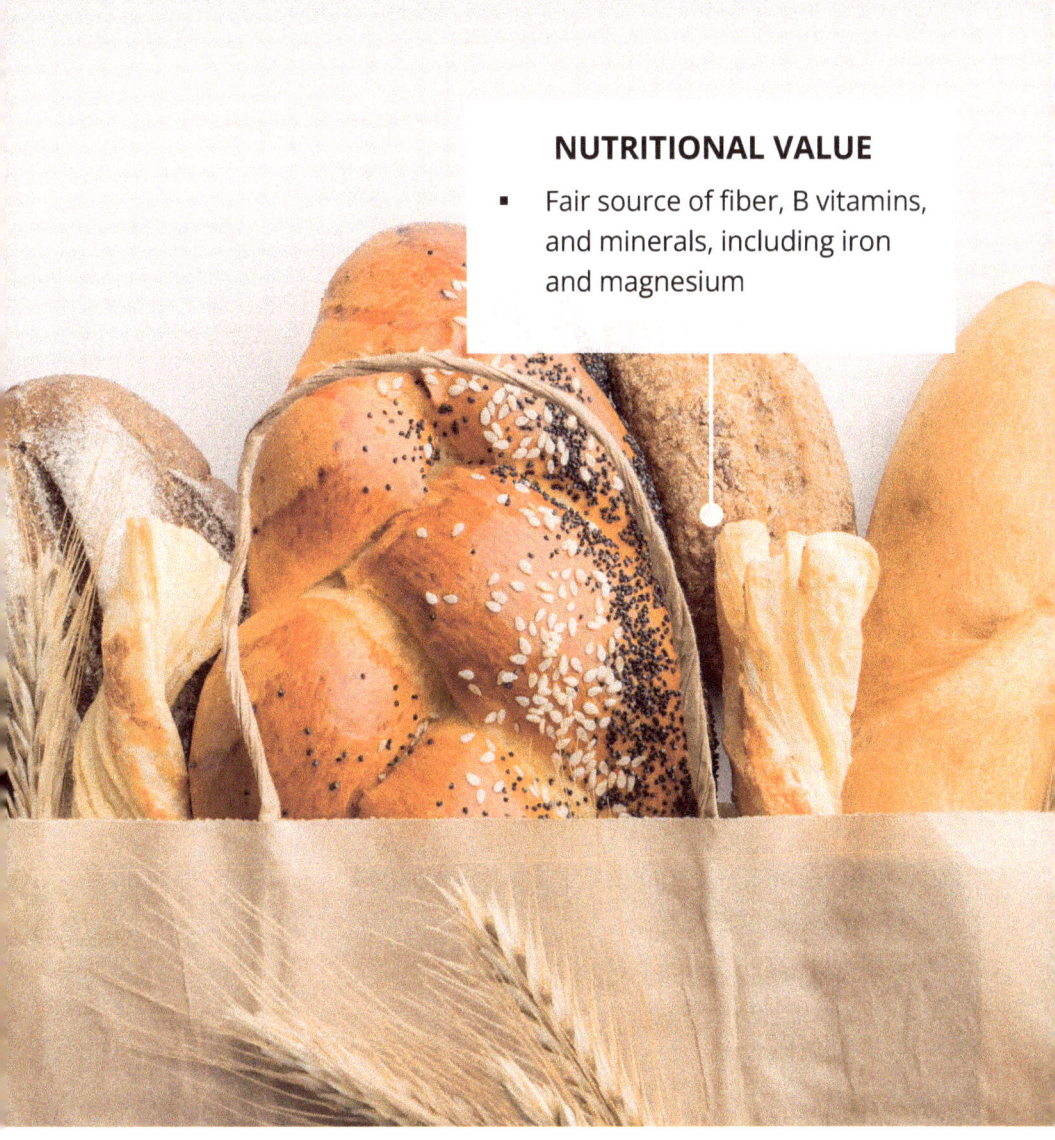

NUTRITIONAL VALUE

- Fair source of fiber, B vitamins, and minerals, including iron and magnesium

35 Wheat

Common Avoidance *Responses*

- Abdominal discomfort
- Gas
- Bloating

Food Clue *Category*

- Poor protein digestion

Food Clue *Explained*

Since gluten is a natural protein commonly found in wheat and other grains, reactions to wheat often suggest difficulty with protein digestion. Gluten reactions can also suggest difficulty with acid breakdown or elimination, or indicate an overload of acid, resulting in an avoidance reaction against eating gluten, since the building blocks of proteins are amino acids.

Profilin protein is another common protein found in many plants that pose a challenge in terms of digestion and absorption.

Allergy *Stats*

- Wheat is considered a top allergen by the National Institute of Health.
- Studies have shown a prevalence of wheat allergy in children of around 0.4 percent, with most showing less reactivity by age twelve.
- Non-celiac gluten sensitivity affects about 6% of the US population.
- Some medical institutes estimate up to eighteen million people in the United States have gluten sensitivity.

HEALTH CONCERNS
- Small intestinal bacterial overgrowth (SIBO)

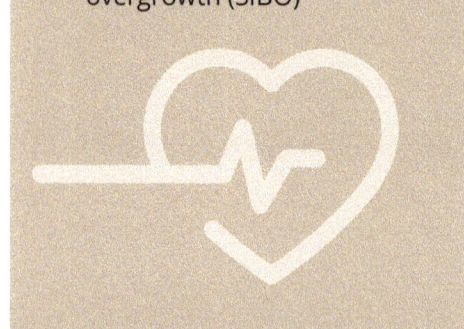
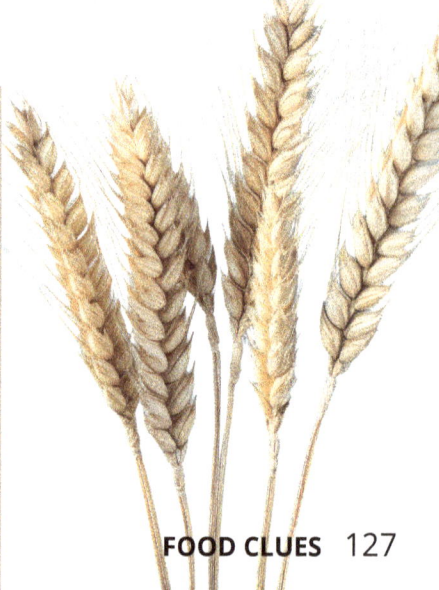

Additional
Information

Gluten reactions commonly occur due to infections, often concentrated in the stomach and small intestine, which disrupt digestion. Gluten reactions could also indicate exposure to acidic chemicals, raising the overall acidity of the body, resulting in avoidance of or reactions to anything acidic.

Allergies to wheat and other foods naturally containing gluten may specifically be in response to the agricultural chemicals used during the growing and preservation processes (e.g., glyphosate).

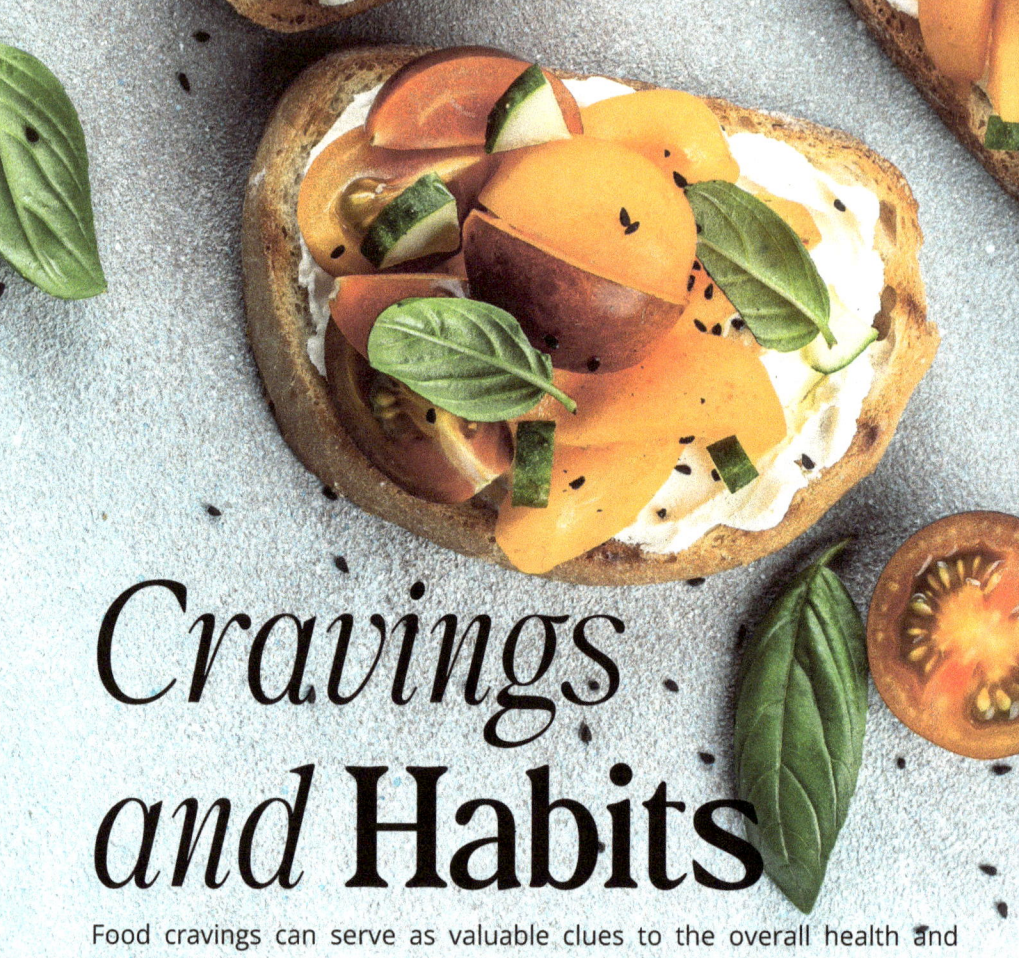

Cravings and Habits

Food cravings can serve as valuable clues to the overall health and functioning of your organs and systems. When your body craves healthy foods like fresh fruits, vegetables, and clean meats, it may indicate issues with digestion and nutrient absorption. In such instances, the body is signaling the need for increased intake to ensure an adequate supply of essential nutrients. Optimizing the processes of digestion, absorption, and nutrient transport becomes crucial for achieving improved health.

On the other hand, cravings for processed foods or those with low nutritional value and empty calories often suggest the presence of an active infection or toxicity, which can specifically affect the nervous system, triggering these specific signals and resulting in such cravings. These instances of cravings are indicative of an underlying imbalance that needs attention and resolution.

Here is a list of ten prevalent food cravings and five common food habits, each linked to potential dysfunctions or infections. Gain a deeper understanding of how your body communicates through these cravings, providing you with the means to decode and address underlying health issues.

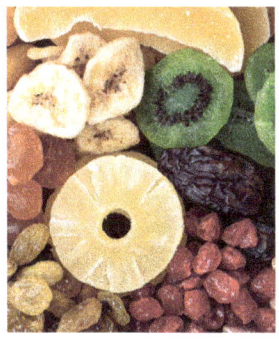

1.

SWEETS: Cravings for sugary foods, whether natural sugars like fruit or processed snacks, often indicate the presence of elevated bacterial levels in the body and likely are related to infection.

2.

FRIED FOODS: Chicken tenders, french fries, potato chips, deep-fried veggies and meats, deep-fried desserts. These cravings often indicate infection by organisms that require fat cells as food or energy sources.

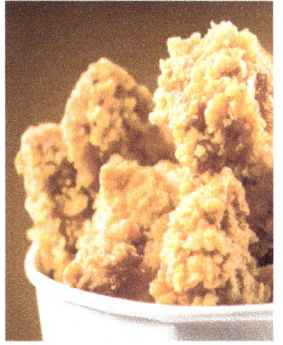

3.

DAIRY PRODUCTS: Milk, cheese, ice cream. These cravings can indicate a need for quick sources of energy through sugar to provide food for infectious organisms, especially bacteria, while still providing minimal energy for organ and system function.

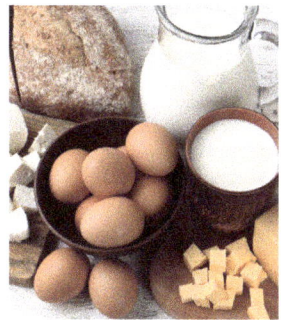

4.

BREAD: Particularly white bread and rolls. Bread can provide sugars to feed bacteria and other infectious organisms but can also be used to balance out bacterial infections by increasing fungal loads in the gut because yeast is a fungus. Even In the presence of an unresolved infection, the body still strives for equilibrium, sometimes allowing the rise of other organisms to maintain gut balance.

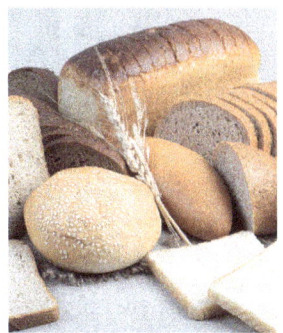

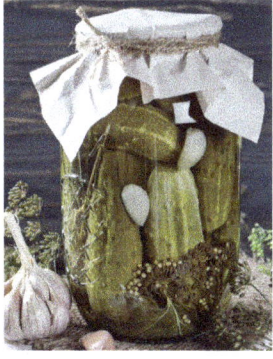

5.

PICKLES: While pickles and pickle juice do contain minerals that can help reduce dehydration, the yellow dye and chemical preservatives in pickles sold to the public reduce the nutritional value of the food due to its processing. In these cases, pickle cravings often indicate the general presence of germs in the body fluids prior to cell invasion, though you cannot specifically know what type of germs by this craving alone. This is because the pickling process involves sugar (which feeds bacteria) and vinegar (which kills viruses, fungi, and parasites).

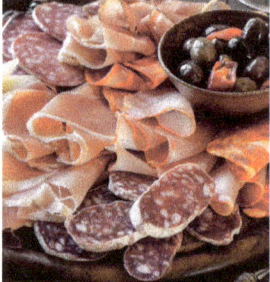

6.
CURED MEATS AND NUTS: These foods are often high in omega-6 fatty acids, which are attractive to bacteria, so these cravings often indicate elevated bacterial loads or actual infection. Common examples include pepperoni, salami, cashews, and walnuts.

7.
MAYONNAISE: Mayo generally has a low nutritional value per serving. Therefore, cravings are generally not associated with a nutrient deficit. However, mayonnaise does contain ethylenediaminetetraacetic acid (EDTA), which is known to eliminate metals from the body. So mayo cravings can be related to the body's need to reduce metal toxicity.

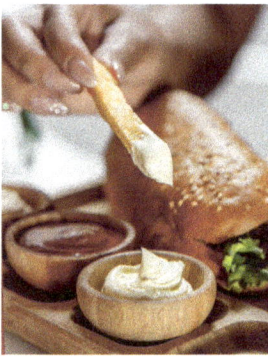

8.
VINEGARY AND SPICY FOODS: Foods with high vinegar or spice content tend to have high acidic properties, which are known to kill viruses, fungi, and other infections, particularly those that are ingested. Stomach acid is a first line of defense against germs that enter the digestive tract. If stomach acid is low, cravings for acidic foods may occur in the presence of an active infection.

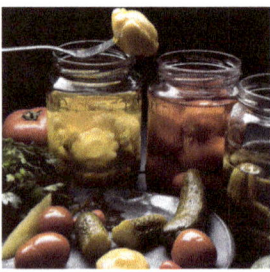

9.
SALT: Salt is a key nutrient that is needed for a number of chemical reactions and functions in the body. Salt cravings can be a clue that the body is having a hard time absorbing, transporting, or using salt. Therefore, the intake of salt will be increased to get the amount it needs despite whatever problem an organ or system may be experiencing.

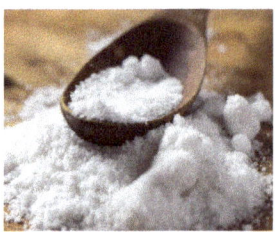

10.
"MOUTH SNACKS": These include ice, mints, gum, and hard candies. Cravings for these types of snacks are often a signal of tongue dysfunction, for example, poor tongue hydration or poor nerve supply to the tongue. Craving mouth snacks can also indicate poor saliva production. Both tongue dysfunction and poor saliva production can cause poor digestion and the development of digestive conditions.

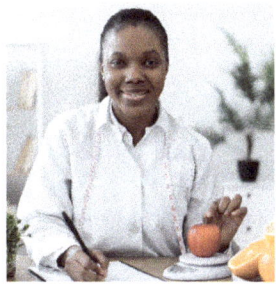

11.

INCREASED APPETITE WITH MINIMAL WEIGHT GAIN: This commonly occurs in instances of significant infection where the invading organism is consuming nearly all the nutrients eaten by the host, leaving little to no nutrients to support organs or body systems. This phenomenon seems to be particularly associated with parasite infections.

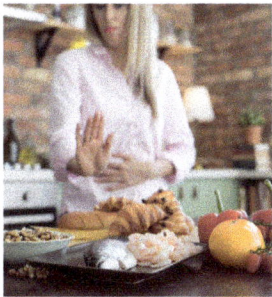

12.

POOR APPETITE: A reduced desire to eat can be associated with general poor digestion. The body will not send signals for you to give it something it doesn't need or can't use. Inflammation, infection, or toxicity can reduce the body's ability to properly digest food and absorb nutrients, resulting in less desire to provide the body with food that it cannot adequately process.

13.

BLOATING BELCHING, AND FLATULENCE: These are common signals of digestive distress. Bloating and belching often stem from the accumulation of gas, triggered by various factors such as rapid food consumption, smoking, or ingesting air while drinking. Gas buildup can also result from undigested food entering the large intestine. When there's a lack of enzymes or communication for effective digestion in the small intestine, the food continues into the large intestine where digeston ocurrs, but in a dysfunctional manner, releasing gas as a byproduct. This introduces the potential for gas buildup and bloating, particularly in the lower abdomen.

14.

FATIGUE AFTER EATING: Fatigue and sleepiness after eating is often a sign of inefficient digestion, which requires more energy to perform and causes the rest of the body to feel sluggish. It can also indicate elevated estrogen levels in the body, as processed foods often contain artificial estrogen-like compounds that are used as preservatives.

15.

PICKY EATING: Picky eating is generally a sign of poor digestion, as you'll tend to gravitate toward foods your body can effectively digest or use effectively for energy. If your picky eating gravitates toward foods high in processed sugar, you may be craving quick sources of energy due to poor digestion or foods to feed an infection. If your food choices include more healthy foods, poor digestion is still a factor to be considered, but without the likelihood of current infection.

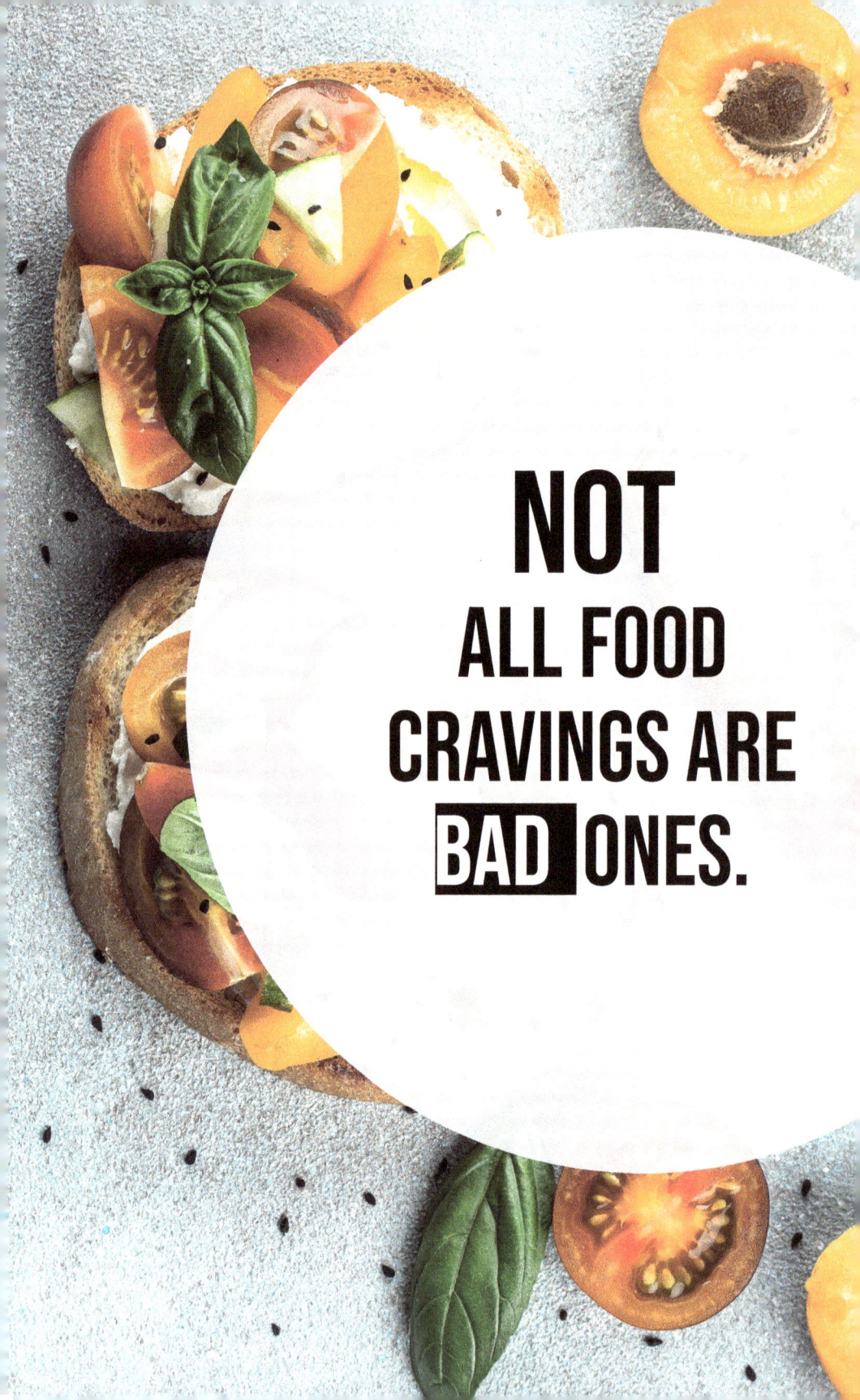

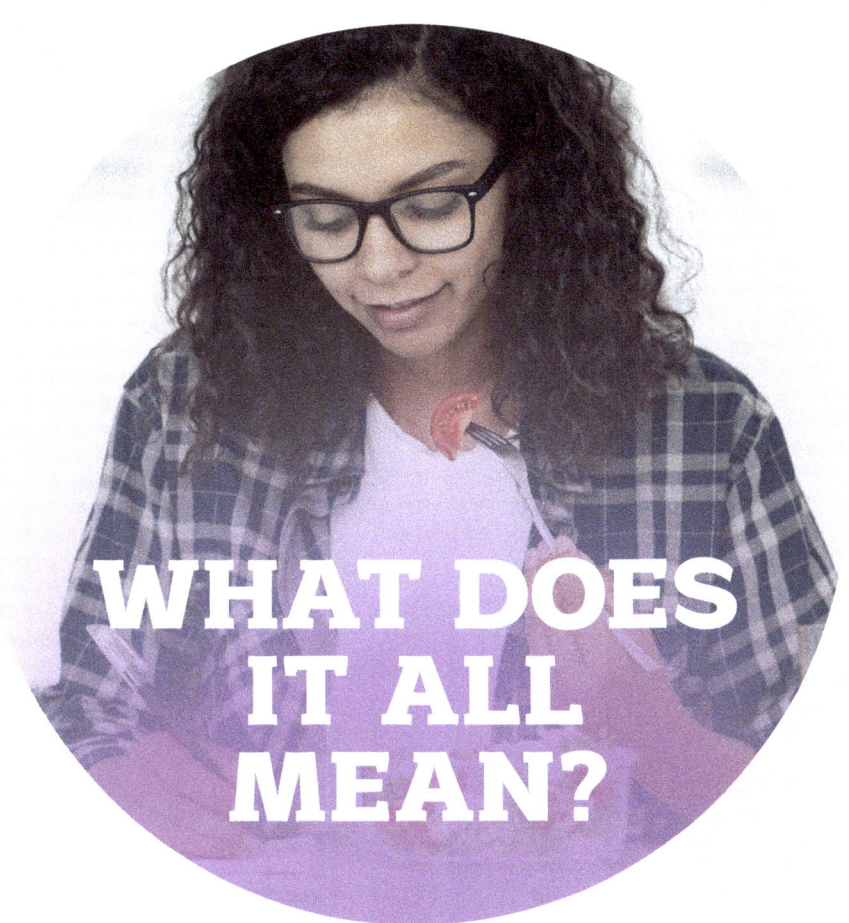

WHAT DOES IT ALL MEAN?

As you've explored the fascinating connections between food dislikes, cravings, and their potential links to various diseases and body issues, it is my hope that you've gained valuable insights into your body's intricate communication with itself through these symptoms. Now, armed with this knowledge, it's time to empower yourself and take proactive steps in your healing journey.

In this next section of the book, I'll present practical strategies and actionable steps that can be taken to leverage your newfound understanding of foods and their impact on your health. By making informed choices and embracing a holistic approach to wellness, you can unlock the path to a healthier, more vibrant life.

Now that you have this information, how do you interpret it all? What does it mean for your health and the opportunity to fully resolve your symptoms and heal your body?

All of this information can be summarized into what I call
The Four Cs: Count, Categories, Concerns and Causes.

Uncover the hidden messages behind your food preferences by utilizing the tally sheets and notes pages in the Food Clues Companion workbook. The workbook was designed to assist you in creating your own Food Clues Wellness Profile, an essential tool for guiding your healing journey. Don't miss out – get your workbook today and take a step towards a healthier and more vibrant you!

Let's begin with the first C, **Count.** As you reviewed the food clues, I'm sure you noticed if any resonated with you. It is crucial to understand that having more clues that relate to you does not signify a worse state of health. A higher number of clues may simply indicate the presence of underlying issues that merit further investigation. If you have been grappling with persistent symptoms, having a greater number of clues could actually be encouraging, as it offers you more opportunities to explore and discover potential recovery solutions.

....

Moving on to **Categories,** the food clue categories provide significant information about why your body is avoiding the foods. Noting these categories offers a deeper perspective on how your organs and systems are being affected as well as your overall health. They can also provide a starting point at which to focus your healing during the early stages of treatment.

....

Next, **Concerns** come into play. When you notice any of the conditions listed in the health concerns section for the foods you avoid, these food clues provide you with valuable context and understanding as to why certain conditions may be present in your life.

....

Lastly, we come to **Causes.** The foods you crave can be valuable indicators, guiding you towards the external causes of any conditions or symptoms you may be struggling with, such as underlying infections or toxicities. Your cravings can serve as messengers, shedding light on the inner workings of your body and offering profound insights into areas that may require attention and healing.

To illustrate this, let's consider an example:

Avoids: avocado, banana, salmon, beans, mushrooms

Picky eater—minimal fresh foods, loves fast food and soda

Cravings: sweets, cured meats, dairy, fried foods, breads

Upon reviewing these cravings and avoidances, you may discover the following:

- Avoiding avocado and mushrooms both point to potential unbalanced gut bacteria levels.
- Common symptoms include gas, bloating and abdominal pain.
- Avoiding bananas, salmon, and beans may indicate difficulties with protein digestion.
- Cravings for sweets, cured meats, and dairy products suggest elevated bacterial loads in the body. The craving for fried foods may be linked to specific "fat-loving" bacteria, and the introduction of a bacteria could be the external cause contributing to the symptoms and issues identified by the foods being avoided.

For someone dealing with digestive, menstrual, or mental health conditions exhibiting these cravings and avoidances, exploring ways to manage bacterial levels in the gut and improve protein digestion could hold promising solutions to reduce symptoms and enhance overall well-being.

Curious to hear how Food Clues helped one of my clients?

Read about Ashleigh's journey as a pre-professional ballet dancer, alleviating her ankle pain just in time for a stellar performance? Scan the QR code to dive into her inspiring story and explore the powerful impact of decoding food clues on her path to healing and peak performance!

When you embrace The Four Cs as your guiding compass on this journey of self-discovery and healing, the wisdom of your food clues will guide your path, leading you toward personalized healing solutions that can foster transformative change and restore balance in your life.

Let these insights be your ally in unlocking the hidden messages behind your food likes and dislikes as you embark on a path of true holistic wellness and nourishment.

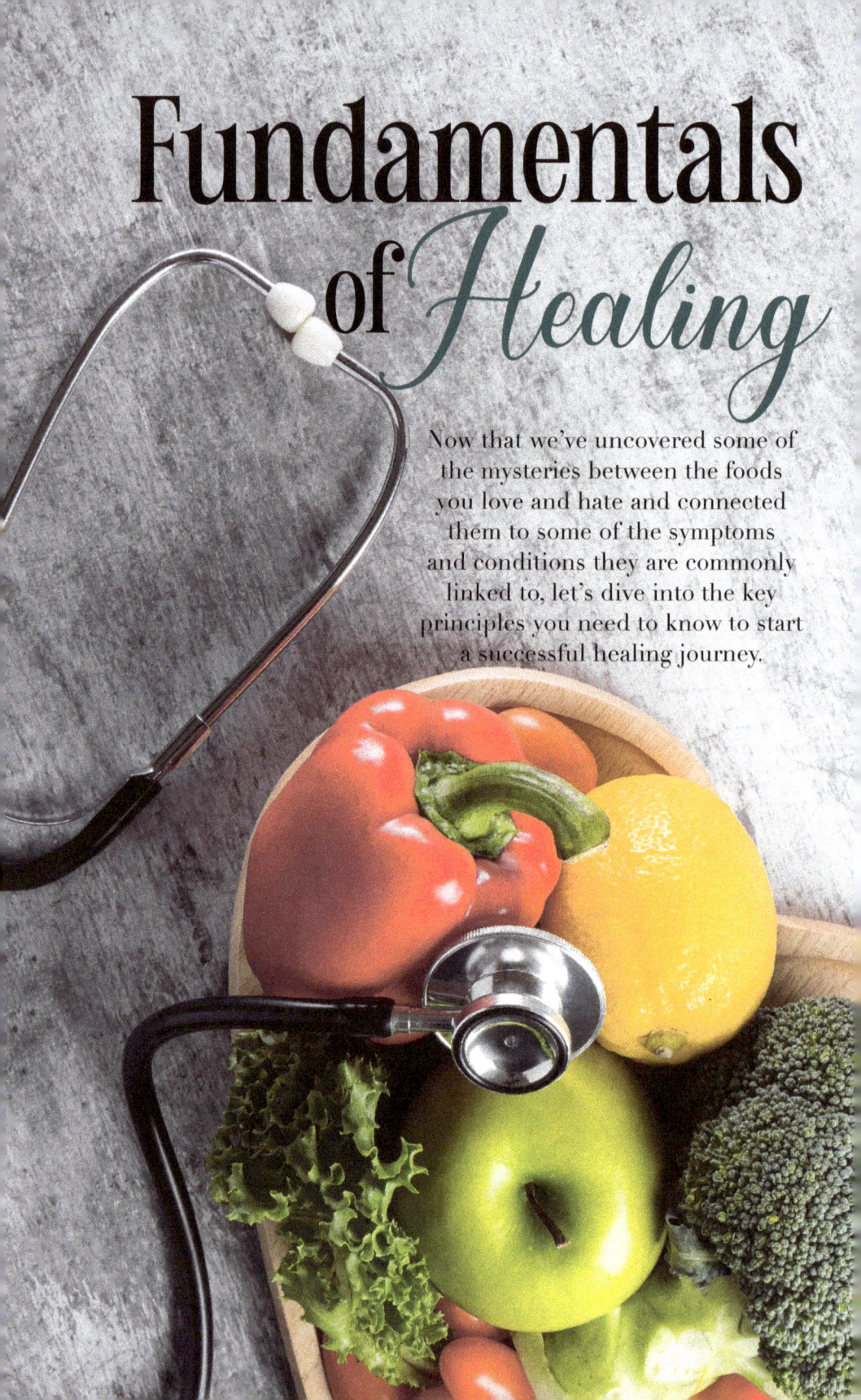

Fundamentals of Healing

Now that we've uncovered some of the mysteries between the foods you love and hate and connected them to some of the symptoms and conditions they are commonly linked to, let's dive into the key principles you need to know to start a successful healing journey.

Understanding root causes

Your body doesn't just wake up and decide not to feel good. Your body doesn't crave disease and illness. Your body doesn't prefer chronic pain and symptoms. So when these things happen, the natural reaction is to wonder how or why they're happening. This is the essence of root cause analysis and healing, which has gotten lots of attention in recent years. While medical and wellness professionals boast that they focus on finding the root cause of your symptoms, many of them miss an extremely important aspect of root cause diagnosis. Here's the secret . . .

Our bodies were designed to be happy and healthy, to stay alive and enjoy life. They were not created to thrive under conditions of illness or disease. If the body never intends to be unwell, that means the cause of illness can't be inside the body. It doesn't make sense for a system that was created to be healthy to spontaneously create an unpleasant environment.

What does that mean? Symptoms and disease occur as the body responds to something it has encountered in the environment. The missing piece to understanding your root cause is this: your true root cause will **always be external** of your body. So if you don't have an answer for your pain, inflammation, disease, or symptom that starts outside of your body, you haven't found your true root cause.

Inflammation isn't your root cause.

Findings in your blood work, imaging, or lab tests are not your root cause.

A disease or condition isn't your root cause.

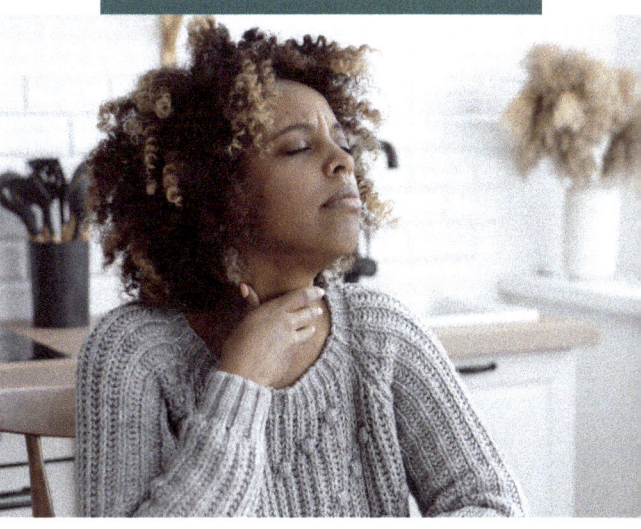

These are all internal reactions from the body in response to an external root cause. Many people haven't resolved their true root cause, or they are still being exposed to it, which often relates to the persistence and sometimes worsening of symptoms. So what are examples of root causes?

The most common external root causes are infection from a living organism, toxicity from non-living substances, and physical trauma, like an accident or injury. In some cases, the eternal cause may include an emotional trauma, causing stress to the brain and nervous system. Stress in the brain can weaken the body's defense, hinder healing, growth, and normal functions crucial for overall health.

Identifying your external root causes is vital to achieving true healing and full resolution of symptoms. Next, you'll need to understand the principles of illness and disease. This will help you understand your current health status and help you monitor your progress better as you move through your healing experience.

How does illness occur?

In general, illness works from simple to complex and from the inside out. Cell damage comes before organ damage, and organ damage comes before system damage. Internal organs, like the liver and large intestine, are often behind unresolved issues of external organs like the skin and eyes.

The infographic below describes my understanding of the disease process after years of studying patterns and symptoms in my clients, and their understanding of the stages of illness has been integral in their healing.

Most people have heard of stages of injury or disease; for example, ankle sprains are described as grade one, two, or three. Cancer and kidney disease are described in stages. I have found that illnesses follow phases as they work their way through the body, and these are the ways I describe those phases to my clients. The external causes that result in illnesses first affect cells and tissues, the more simple structures in the body. As they grow and spread, they affect more complex organs and body systems.

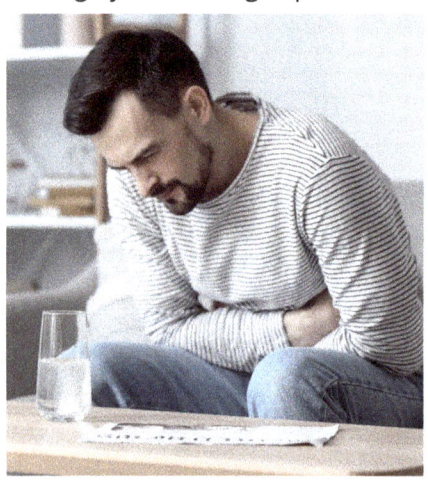

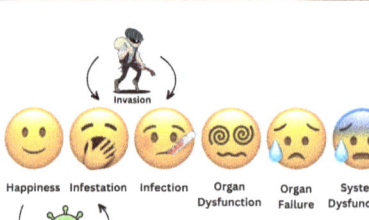

FOOD CLUES 139

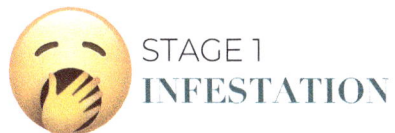

STAGE 1
INFESTATION

This occurs immediately after an infectious organism or toxin has been introduced into the body through exposure and mostly involves body fluids. The presence of infestation in the blood and body fluids reduces the ability to deliver oxygen and other nutrients to the body's organs and tissues. It also reduces the ability for waste to be removed from the body and properly eliminated. This slows down many of the body's processes and reduces their overall performance, which is why the key symptom of infestation is generalized fatigue.

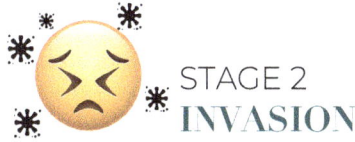

STAGE 2
INVASION

After an infection has consumed all the nutrients and resources it can, or a toxin has broken down through the majority of vessel structures, focus turns to cells of other organs and tissues. In the case of infections, organisms start to "break in" to cells of tissues and organs. This is often where you start to see signs of inflammation, particularly pain and swelling in the affected area. While many are familiar with pain and swelling when it has to do with muscles, bones, and joints, pain and swelling can occur in any tissue or organ and often relates to common musculoskeletal issues that are not resolved with interventions, like exercise or medication. For example, a swollen liver is often responsible for changes in rib and shoulder position, like having one shoulder higher than the other or one side of the ribcage more forward than the other. People are often ticklish or tender around the ribcage when the liver is swollen.

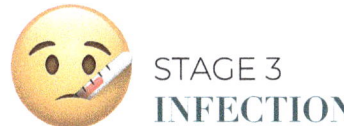

STAGE 3
INFECTION

This stage is marked by a significant breakdown of cell function as organisms that have broken in begin to consume the cell's resources, like fats and proteins. The effects on the cell trigger an aggressive immune response, which is why the key symptoms of infection are fever, chills, or allergy symptoms, based on the type of organism involved.

All of these stages can occur in order or occur at the same time, causing you to experience multiple symptoms as organisms grow and continue to consume the resources meant for your cells.

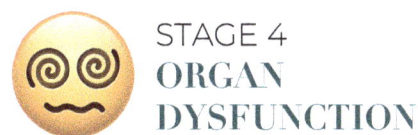

STAGE 4
ORGAN DYSFUNCTION

As the infection of cells continues, it begins to affect the involved organ. Stage 4, organ dysfunction, sets in as a given organ is still able to perform its tasks but does so in a disorderly or erratic matter. For example, dysfunction of the heart would include changes in heart rate and rhythm, such as atrial fibrillation or A-fib. Muscle or joint pain around the dysfunctional organ is common, along with swelling and repeated injury in the nearby area.

As infection or toxicity continue to break down an organ, **organ failure** can occur (e.g., heart failure, heart attack). Finally, organ failure can affect the performance of its involved system, creating system dysfunction and failure, which corresponds to the diagnosis and progression of diseases. In severe cases, prolonged system dysfunction and failure may result in death.

Once you find the external root cause, examining your symptoms may provide clues related to the organs and systems most involved. Your food clues may be able to help you connect your symptoms to the problematic areas, now that you know what they can mean.

Understanding your symptoms and stage of illness can also help you monitor your progress. For example, if you started your healing journey with brain fog, fatigue, joint pain, and irregular menstrual cycles, it's likely you were experiencing some organ failure (e.g., ovaries) and some system dysfunction (e.g., reproductive system).

If you've experienced improvements in your menstrual cycle and reduced pain after a couple of months, but fatigue and brain fog persist, it could indicate that the illness has been eliminated from most organs and tissues. However, it may still be present in the blood and body fluids, signifying an ongoing infestation phase..

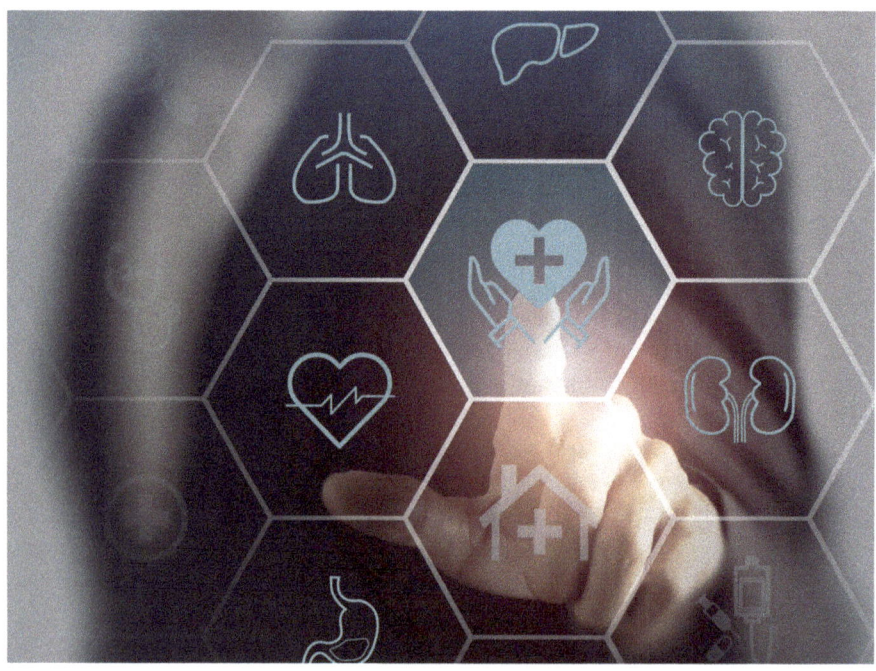

How does the body prioritize healing from a condition or disease?

Knowing how the body prioritizes healing will help you keep your expectations realistic when tackling your health. To start, the body prioritizes healing opposite to how it's experienced in most cases. Some practitioners call this the hierarchy of function, based on the importance of the body's systems and how they contribute to everyday living. I prefer to call it the hierarchy of dysfunction because this perspective seems to speak better to the client with symptoms they can't heal or resolve.

In short, many of us experience our symptoms closer to the top of the pyramid in less dominant systems. These are systems that are important but not absolutely crucial for biological tasks that keep you alive (e.g., brain function, circulation). The top of the pyramid is where we see and feel the symptoms of the condition or disease. However, in most cases, the reason symptoms aren't resolving is because the primary location of the issue causing the condition or disease is toward the bottom of the pyramid.

This is not to be confused with a root cause, because we're still dealing with what's inside the body, and root causes are always external. But this can shed some light on why your symptoms may not be resolving if you're focusing on treatments that involve the areas closer to the top of the pyramid. If you have symptoms there, it's highly likely that the cause is also affecting the lower half of the pyramid where the more dominant systems lie. You will definitely need to address those areas and systems for full healing and recovery of symptoms to occur.

Hair
Skin
Teeth

Muscle
Fascia/Joint

Endocrine
(Hormones)

Organs

Nerves

Vascular

Gut

Lymphatic

Brain Stress (physical/emotional)

Putting it all Together

As we bring together all the insights and knowledge we have explored so far regarding identifying and understanding food clues, let's consider how you can effectively approach your symptoms and embark on a new path to healing:

First and foremost, take a closer look at the patterns that emerge within the food clue categories, avoidance symptoms, and potential causes found in your food clues. Notice how many of these overlap across the foods you avoid.

Remember, your root cause investigation should not come to a halt until you have traced the cause of your symptoms to a factor external to your body. Identifying and addressing external causes is paramount to achieving sustainable healing and lasting relief.

In addition, pay close attention to your symptoms, as they can provide valuable insights into the stage of illness you might be experiencing. Understanding the stage of illness can guide your treatment decisions and help you prioritize areas that need immediate attention.

As you seek understanding of how your food clues relate to your overall health, consider the role of dominant body systems in influencing your symptoms. Even if you perceive the effects in less dominant systems, consider how they may be influenced by the more prominent ones. All aspects of your body's intricate systems are interconnected, and addressing the more dominant systems will likely hold the potential to alleviate symptoms in other areas as well.

By considering these essential points, you will be better equipped to navigate your healing journey with clarity and purpose. Your dedication to exploring the hidden messages behind your food likes and dislikes, and understanding their significance, lays the foundation for a renewed sense of well-being. As you take these steps, may you feel empowered in your pursuit of holistic health and embark on a path of true healing. Remember, every individual's journey is unique, and I encourage you to embrace your personal experience and celebrate each step forward on your path to wellness.

Using food as clues vs food as medicine

Understanding how your body accepts and processes food can provide powerful insights into your overall health and potential for healing. You may have come across the familiar adage, "Food is medicine," and indeed, it holds truth. However, let's dive deeper into this concept to shed more light on its significance.

The true potential of food as medicine, offering solutions for managing illness and disease, is fully optimized when your body systems are healthy and functioning without significant deficits. In this state, healing nutrients from food can be effectively broken down, absorbed, and transported to areas of your body that require support and healing. This is especially true for the digestive system which plays a pivotal role in unlocking the nutritional and health benefits that food has to offer.

However, when the digestive system is impaired or compromised, digestion, absorption, and nutrient transport may be hindered, resulting in minimal or negligible

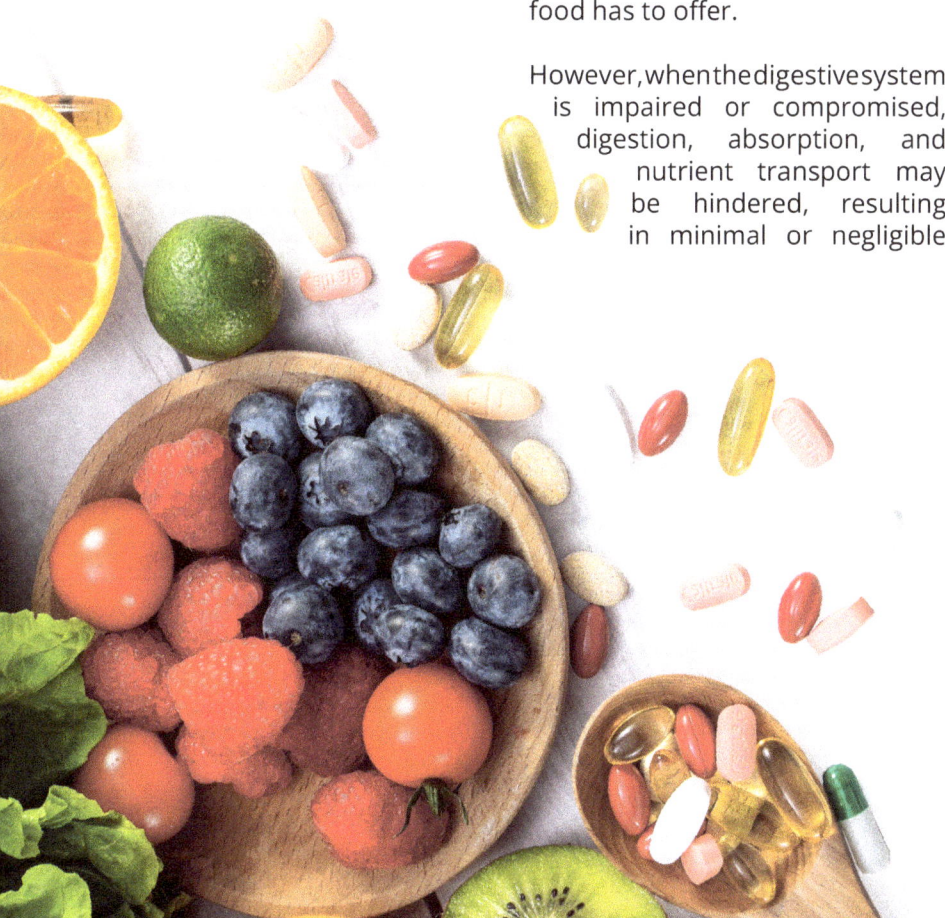

benefits from the food you consume. In fact, your body may even reject certain healing foods if the digestive system is unable to handle them effectively. This may explain why some fruits and vegetables, which are supposed to be good for you, are included in this book. Their avoidance often points to an underlying digestive issue.

Thus, it is essential to recognize that avoiding healthy foods could be an indicator of difficulties with digestion or elimination. Such patterns of avoidance may reveal valuable clues about your digestive health and help pinpoint areas that require attention and healing. On the other hand, cravings for less healthy foods can also offer significant clues about potential infections or toxicities in your body. These cravings can be a symptom of underlying issues contributing to the avoidance of healthier food choices.

By paying close attention to your body's responses to different foods, you can discover a ton of insights into your well-being. Embracing these food clues and understanding their significance empowers you to make informed choices for your health and well-being. So as you embark on your healing journey, remember to be mindful of how your body interacts with various foods. Embrace the wisdom that your food choices hold and let them guide you toward optimal health and vitality.

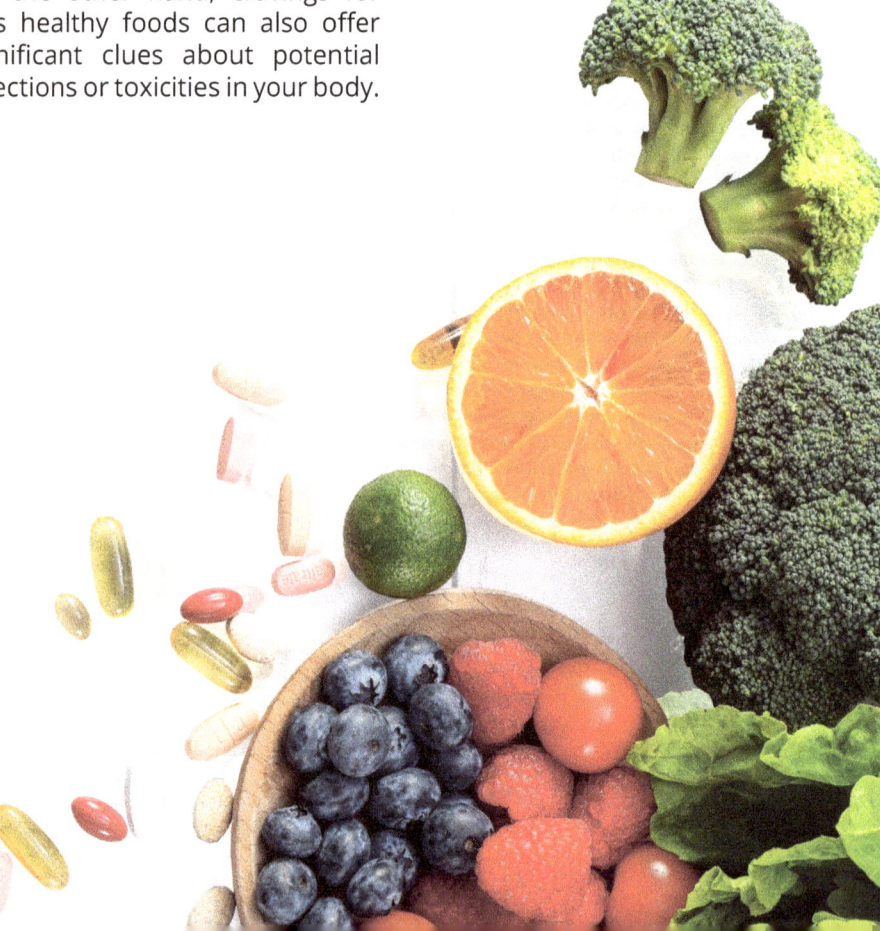

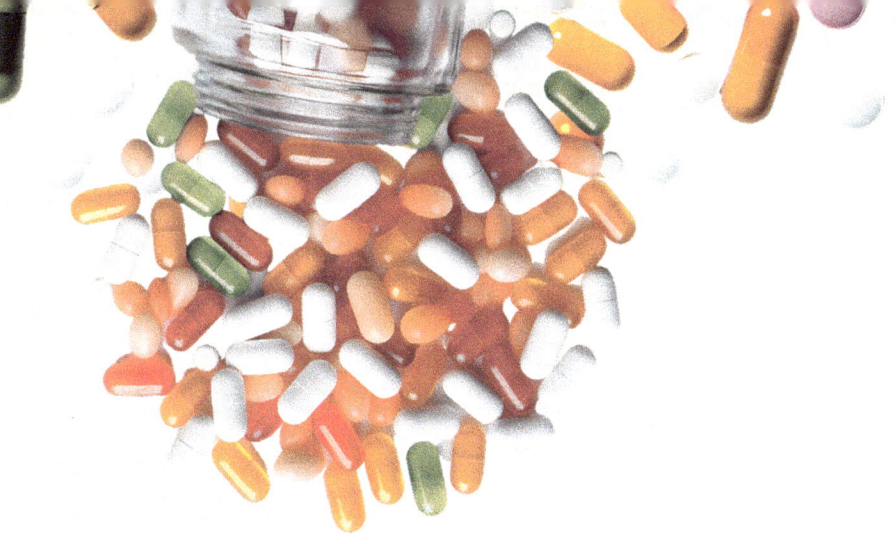

The doctor of the **FUTURE** will no longer treat the **HUMAN FRAME** with drugs, but rather will cure and prevent disease with **NUTRITION.**

~ Thomas Edison

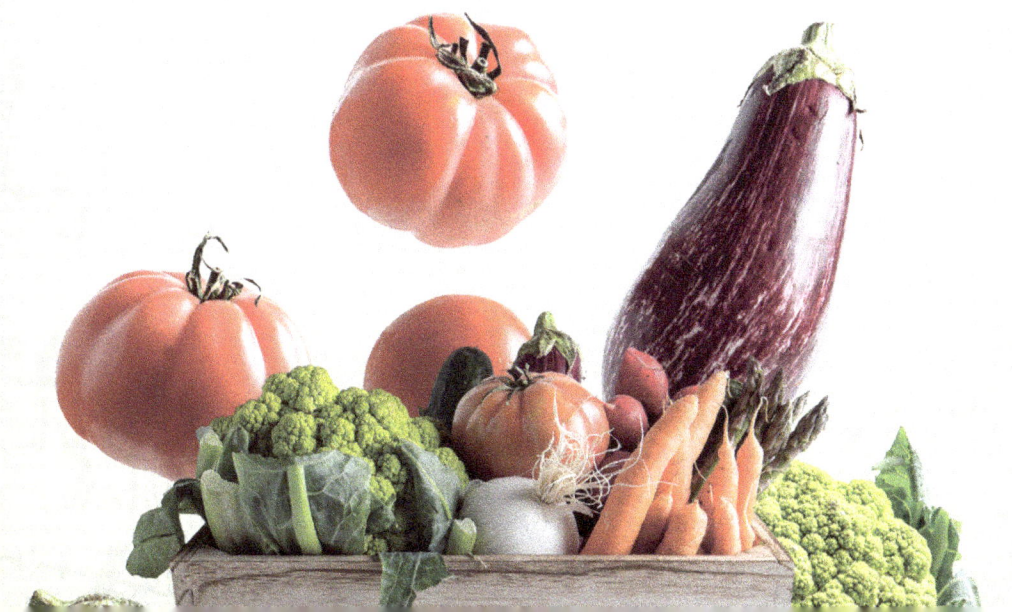

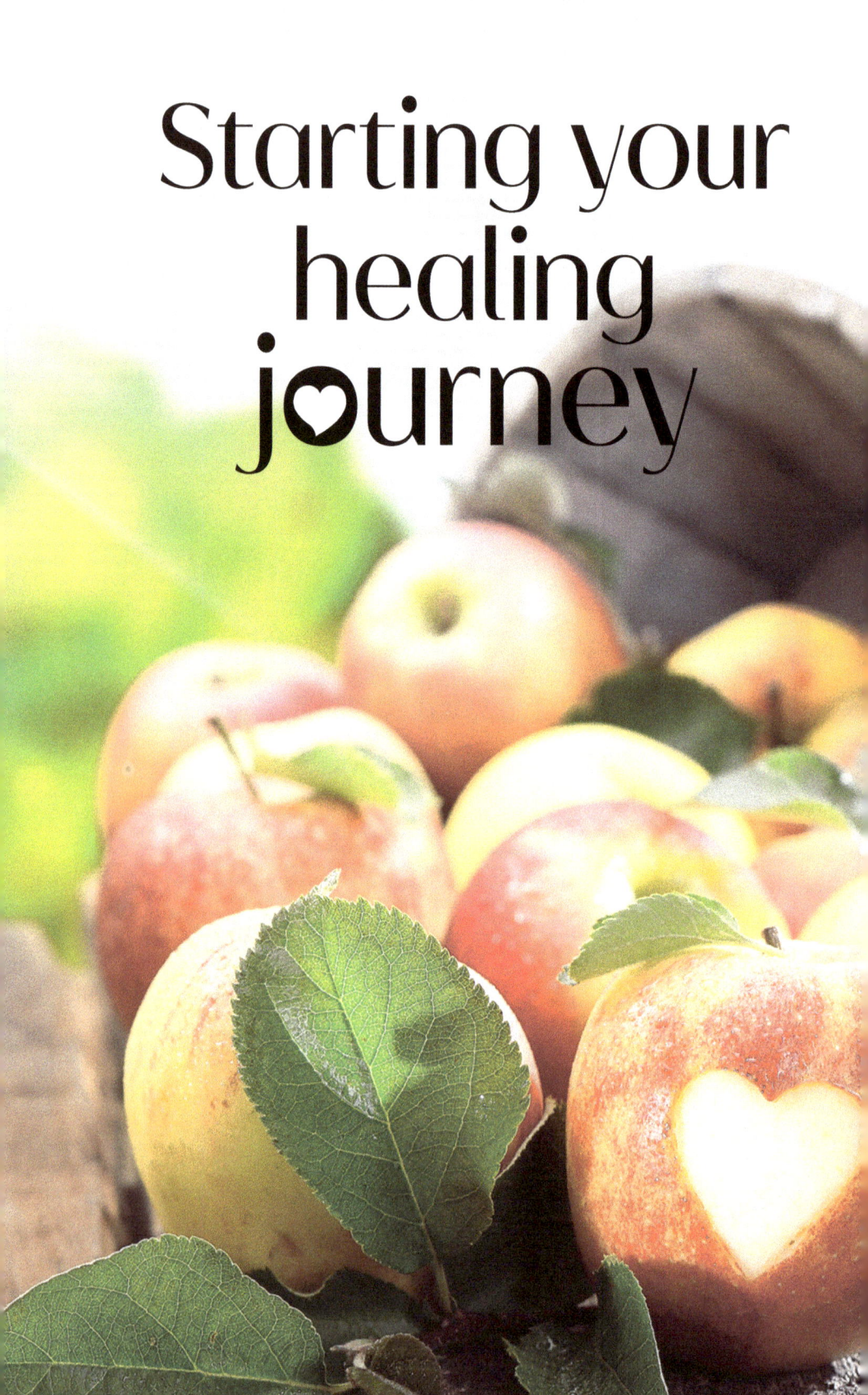

Starting your healing journey

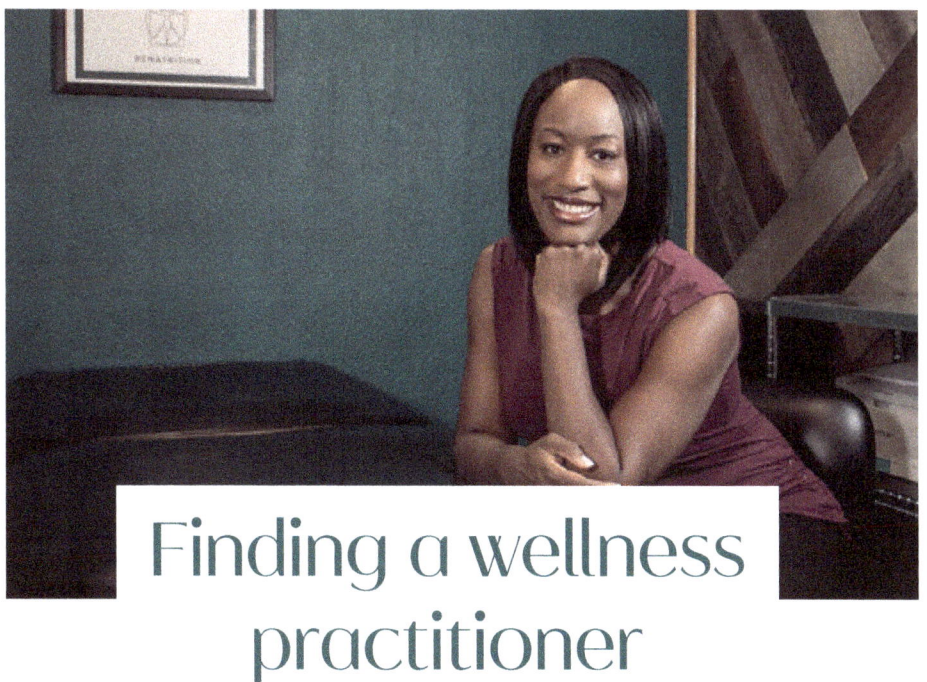

Finding a wellness practitioner

Just like finding the right pair of jeans that fits you perfectly, the search for the ideal wellness practitioner can be both empowering and fulfilling. Whether you're seeking a doctor, therapist, nutritionist, or any other health specialist, this process is all about finding a partner in your well-being journey.

Next, we'll explore the essential factors to consider, the questions to ask, and the signs that indicate you've discovered a practitioner who will not only support your health goals but also make you feel seen, heard, and valued as a unique individual.

In the quest for the perfect wellness practitioner, there are some crucial steps to take to ensure you find someone who truly understands and supports your health goals. First and foremost, tapping into the power of your personal network can yield valuable insights. Don't hesitate to seek referrals from family or friends, as their firsthand experiences can provide you with valuable guidance.

Explore social media platforms to ensure a practitioner's approach to treatment includes finding and eliminating external root causes. It's vital to find someone who goes beyond mere symptom management, aiming for holistic healing solutions that target the underlying causes of health challenges.

An essential aspect to consider is how much emphasis the practitioner places on food as a vital treatment tool. You now understand that merely avoiding certain foods won't lead to true healing. Look for someone who views food in the right context, incorporating it strategically to foster your well-being.

Beyond qualifications and approaches, connecting with a wellness practitioner who aligns with your values and resonates with you is equally crucial. Take into account factors like age, gender, and overall energy, as these elements can influence the relationship with your clinician.

Once you've narrowed down your options and decided to schedule a consultation, take the opportunity to assess how much time the practitioner devotes to listening. Openly share your most pressing concerns and gauge their receptivity and attentiveness.

Furthermore, observe how inquisitive they are about your current health status and feelings regarding your well-being. A practitioner who asks thoughtful questions often has a genuine interest in understanding your unique circumstances.

Don't shy away from discussing past experiences with other treatment programs or practitioners that may have fallen short for you. Pay close attention to their response, as it will reveal their ability to adapt their approach to your specific needs.

Lastly, clarity is key. Ensure you fully comprehend how they plan to help you overcome your health challenges. Transparency in their approach will give you the confidence to embark on this healing journey together.

Remember, finding the right wellness practitioner is about building a partnership that fosters trust, understanding, and effective collaboration. Go with your gut (pun fully intended) and pick the practitioner that resonates with you the most and truly gives you the sense that they will do all in their power to help you achieve the healing you deserve.

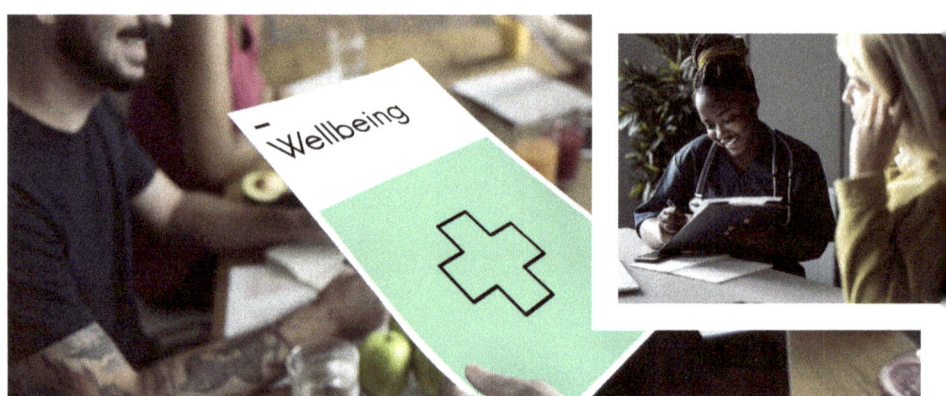

An overview of Renatrition's Food Clues Total Healing Program

Now that we have explored the process of finding the right wellness practitioner, let's delve into the heart of my holistic health treatment framework. This framework has been carefully designed over the years to successfully address chronic health issues and resolve symptoms for good.

The journey begins with the **Cleanse Phase,** where our primary focus is to maximize the liver's performance, the body's chief detox organ. By cleaning and strengthening the pathways between the liver and exit points for toxins, such as the colon and the bladder, we pave the way for future phases of the program, where infections and toxicities can be efficiently eliminated from your system.

In the **Eradicate & Eliminate Phase,** we tackle the direct elimination of infections and other biological illnesses from your body. We also take special care to ensure that your lymph nodes and vessels, which help remove wastes from your body, are clean and strong enough to support the liver's job of detoxification. Drawing from your medical history and assessment findings, we create a personalized plan to target and eliminate these sources of imbalance. During this phase we also focus on clearing toxins, excess hormones and acids along with any other unwanted substances to create a clean slate for healing and restoration.

Moving forward, the **Repair Phase** emphasizes the healing and regrowth of damaged tissues, organs, and systems caused by infections, overload, or toxicity. This phase nurtures the body's inherent capacity for regenerating and revitalizing its essential components, paving the way for a renewed sense of wellness.

With the foundation of healing laid, focus turns toward the **Optimization Phase,** dedicated to fine-tuning your organ and system performance. Here, we aim to bring target tissues, substances, organs, and systems to 100% efficiency using a blend of nutrient support, neurological guidance and retraining, and lifestyle and mindset training. The goal is to ensure that your body operates at its peak potential at all times.

For those seeking further enhancement in their daily activities, hobbies, or athletic performances, the **Performance Phase** focuses on customized conditioning exercises, carefully selected to improve neuromotor performance and align with your specific desired activities.

Throughout this transformative journey, careful attention is given to the order of the phases, recognizing the critical role of efficient waste elimination that is needed before infection management and tissue healing can occur. Adequate waste removal is often underestimated, and its significance lies in preventing waste backup and potential complications that can arise from incomplete digestion. Ensuring proper elimination is also vital in managing and removing toxins and infections from organs and tissues, avoiding reabsorption, and preventing new symptoms and dysfunction.

With this comprehensive treatment framework, my goal is to guide you toward optimal well-being, addressing not just the symptoms, but the underlying causes of health challenges. When you embrace each phase of this journey with care and commitment, you'll discover a newfound sense of vitality and balance, empowering you to live life to the fullest with renewed joy and wellness.

Not only will you experience a transformative restoration of your well-being through the Renatrition Healing Framework, but you will also come away with a wealth of knowledge and a deeper understanding of the spectrum of exposure, illness, and healing. Armed with this newfound wisdom, you will be better equipped to respond appropriately in the future when new symptoms or injuries arise.

So alongside the tangible improvements in your health, expect to emerge from your Renatrition experience with a newfound sense of empowerment and a deeper appreciation of your body's innate healing abilities. For instance, you'll comprehend the role of a fever, recognizing its positive aspects and its implications for immune system function. This knowledge will help alleviate unnecessary panic when you or a loved one experiences it. Armed with this valuable understanding, you'll confidently navigate symptoms in the future with the tools and knowledge you've gained.

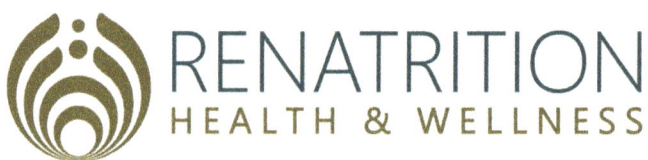

Food Allergy Total Freedom Program

Do specific food allergies or intolerances hold you back from living the life you desire?

Food Allergy Total Freedom Program is a transformative journey designed to empower you with the ability to eat without restrictions. The mission of the program is to "be free to eat what you want, when you want, where you want, fearlessly."

Who is it for?

- **Seekers of True Freedom:** Those who believe in the possibility of eliminating food allergies and desire the freedom to eat without restrictions.

- **Wellness Wisdom Seekers:** Individuals seeking knowledge and understanding of their body's responses and the purpose of recommended treatments.

- **Food Allergy Freedom Fighters:** Committed individuals ready for the healing journey, understanding that it takes time and dedication.

What's included?

- **Informative Videos** explaining body functions, the impact on allergies, and detailed protocols.

- **Protocol Review Videos** outlining the specific protocols, solutions, purposes, and troubleshooting tips.

- **Weekly Group Coaching Calls** to seek guidance and support throughout the process.

- **Facebook Group** for connection and community support with others in the program.

- **Supplements** that have been personally tested and included, no additional costs.

- **Diet Options** that complement vegetarian or vegan lifestyles.

What's the next step?

Apply to the Food Allergy Total Freedom Program and embark on your journey to freedom from food allergies.

Want to work with me?

At Renatrition, I've redesigned the healing journey to address the core factors hindering your progress. Utilizing my distinctive framework, we go beyond treating infections and toxins. We start with a vital external root cause analysis, followed by thorough cleansing and optimization of your body's detoxification capabilities. I've poured my heart into understanding the body's intricacies, dedicating years to mastering the art of holistic healing. With this knowledge, I created a program that gives clients the relief they've been searching for that eludes them when they focus on reducing symptoms and managing their condition or disease.

What does it look like to work with me?

Your journey with Renatrition is designed to fit seamlessly into your busy life. It's about simplicity—a daily five-minute supplement regimen that I've meticulously curated for quality and affordability. This partnership is all about supporting you, from our treatment sessions to those in-between moments when questions arise.

You could venture down this healing road on your own, but why not make it smoother? With your Renatrition program, you're investing in peace of mind. I've done the research and handpicked the best supplements, so you don't have to worry about quality. When symptoms pop up, I'll be right there, deciphering the healing process so you can relax and trust it—dosages, delivery method, and usage, all catered to you for maximum efficiency. If you have difficulty swallowing capsules, I have options for you. If you are vegetarian, I have options for you. If you have sensitive skin, I have options for you.

What sets Renatrition apart is my multifaceted approach to healing. Your path is unique, and that's where my toolbox of various modalities is critical. Vitamins, essential oils, herbal supplements, thermal camera imaging, hands-on lymphatic techniques, corrective exercise, and more come into play. It's a blend that caters to your needs, fostering healing on all levels.

So if you're ready to take that step toward renewed vitality and balance with me, I invite you to connect. Let's discuss how a Renatrition program can be your partner in your personal health journey. Schedule a chat session at https://renatrition.com/letschat today. Your well-being deserves this investment, and together, we'll carve out a path that's uniquely yours.

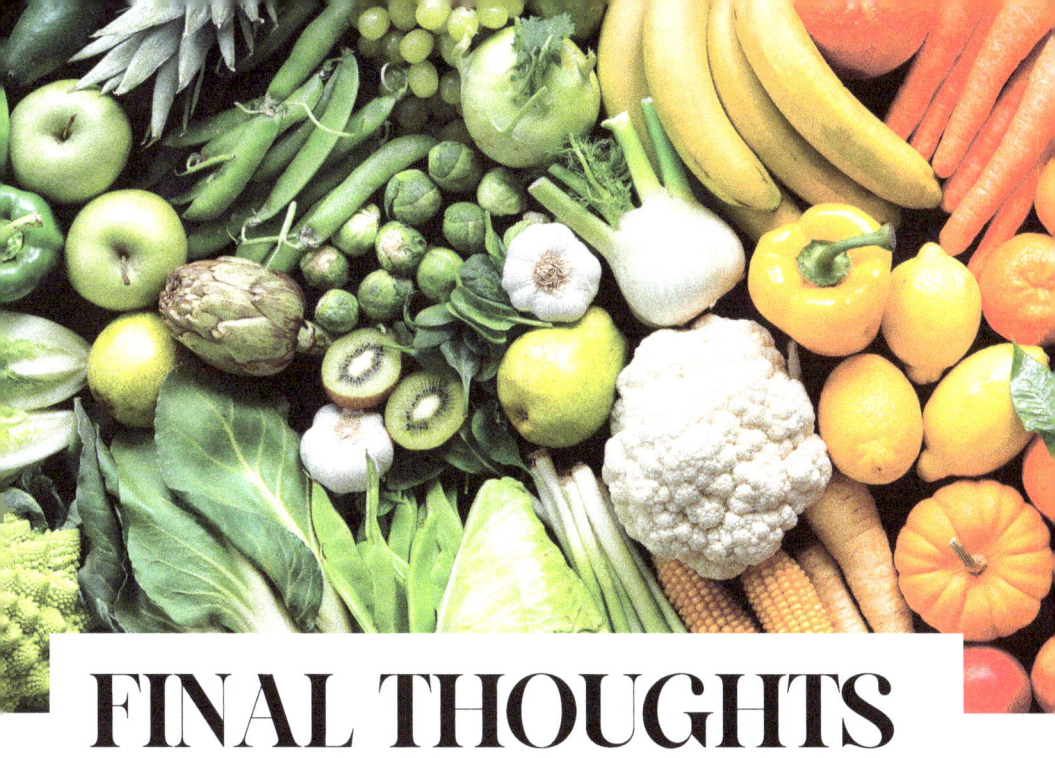

FINAL THOUGHTS

As you reach the end of this journey through the world of food clues, I sincerely hope that you have found invaluable insights and revelations that resonate with you on a profound level. My greatest wish is that you feel empowered and equipped with simple yet potent tools to better understand the subtle details of your health.

This book has been a labor of love, driven not only by a passion for deciphering the hidden messages within our food likes and dislikes but also by a calling to guide others toward genuine healing solutions. It goes beyond the suppression of symptoms for temporary relief and delves into the realm of true holistic wellness.

Throughout these pages, my aim has been to educate and empower you with practical knowledge to help you take ownership of your health journey. You do not need a medical degree to comprehend the essentials of human health and the foundations of illness and disease. My vision for the future of healthcare revolves around fostering a sense of autonomy within each individual, where you can confidently make informed decisions about your health, the treatments you choose, and the practitioners you partner with. Now is the moment to break free from blindly adhering to "doctor's orders" or media recommendations without comprehending their true purpose or implications.

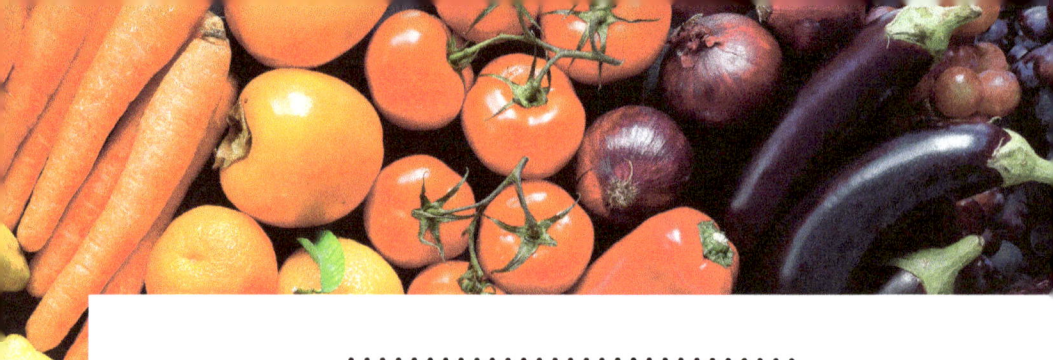

. . . .

I have a friend who is known for repeatedly saying something like, "Owning a business is the personal development course you never knew you signed up for." I believe writing a book is the same. The experience of writing Food Clues has been a journey of courage and vulnerability, building my resilience in the face of criticism and opposition. It has also acted as a transformative springboard, propelling me toward newfound opportunities for personal growth, professional visibility, and the profound privilege of helping others.

Through Food Clues, I have found my authentic voice within the Western healthcare system. This book stands as a firm expression of my beliefs and convictions, a testament of how I view health and healing. My desire is to inspire a paradigm shift, fostering a profound change in how people approach and cherish their well-being by giving power back to the client.

As we part ways, may the knowledge you've gleaned from these pages serve as a compass on your path toward optimal health. Embrace the wisdom of your food clues, for they carry a unique language waiting to be deciphered by each of us individually. May you embrace your personal journey of self-discovery and healing, forging ahead with confidence, grace, and the profound understanding that you possess the innate power to transform your health and life.

My ultimate hope for you, as you conclude this book, is to firmly believe that true healing and freedom from food allergies, intolerances, and their associated symptoms is possible.

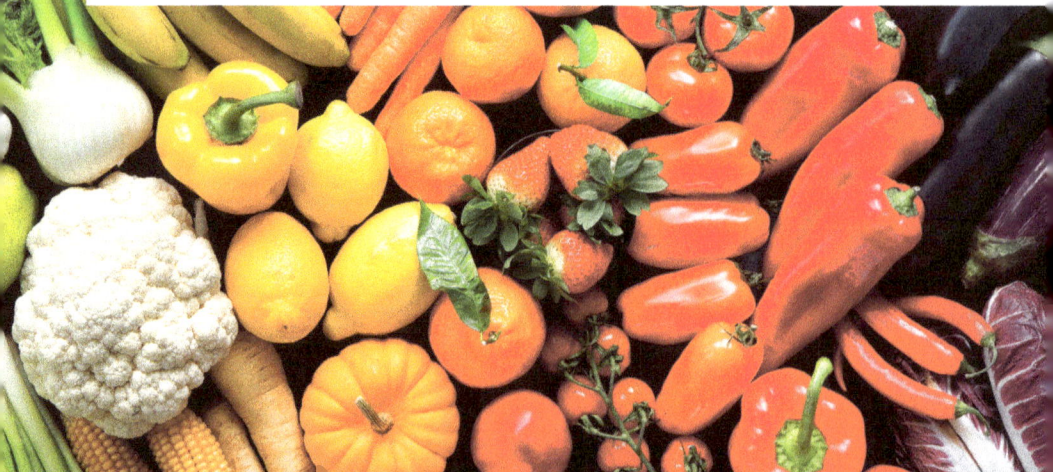

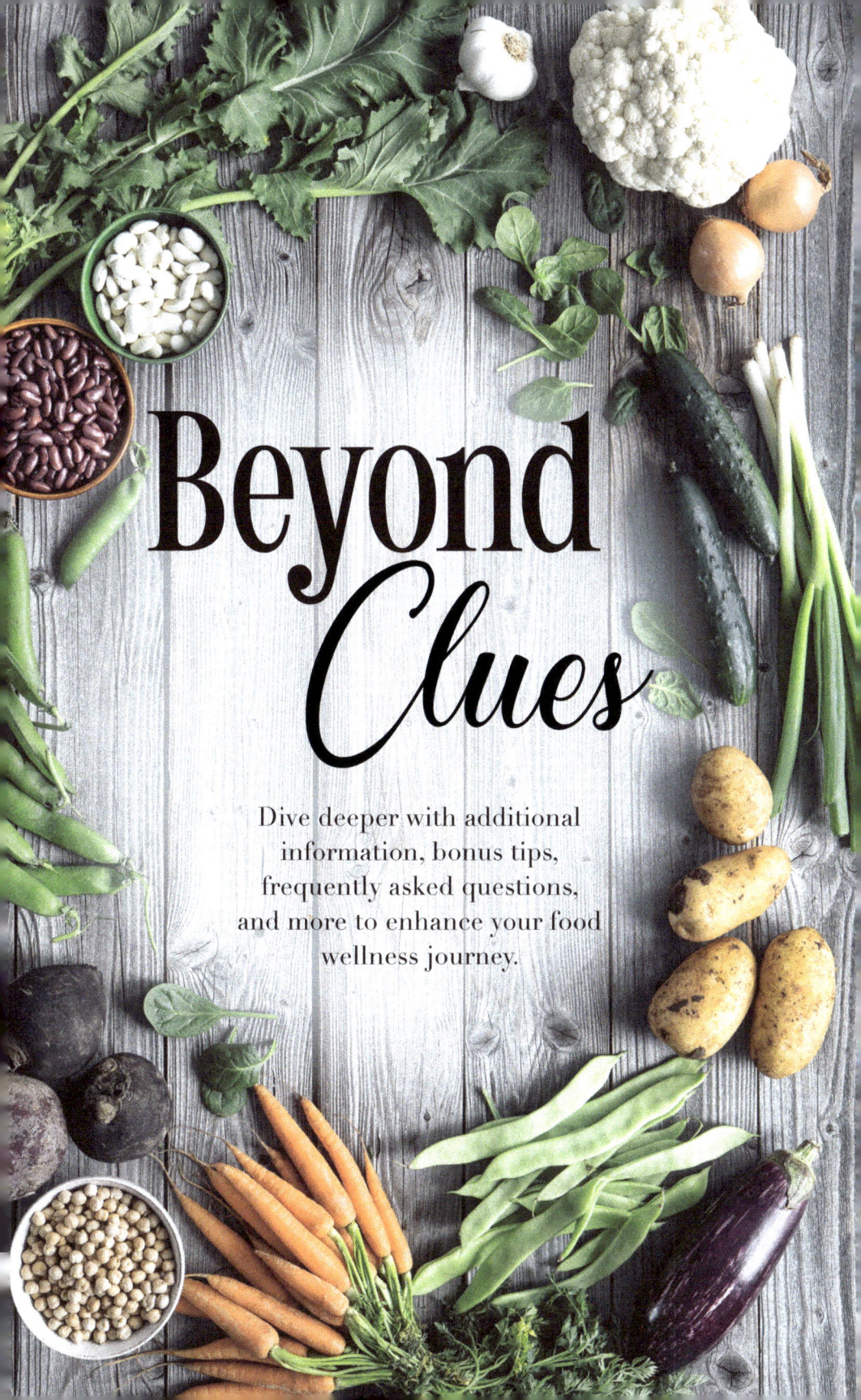

Beyond Clues

Dive deeper with additional information, bonus tips, frequently asked questions, and more to enhance your food wellness journey.

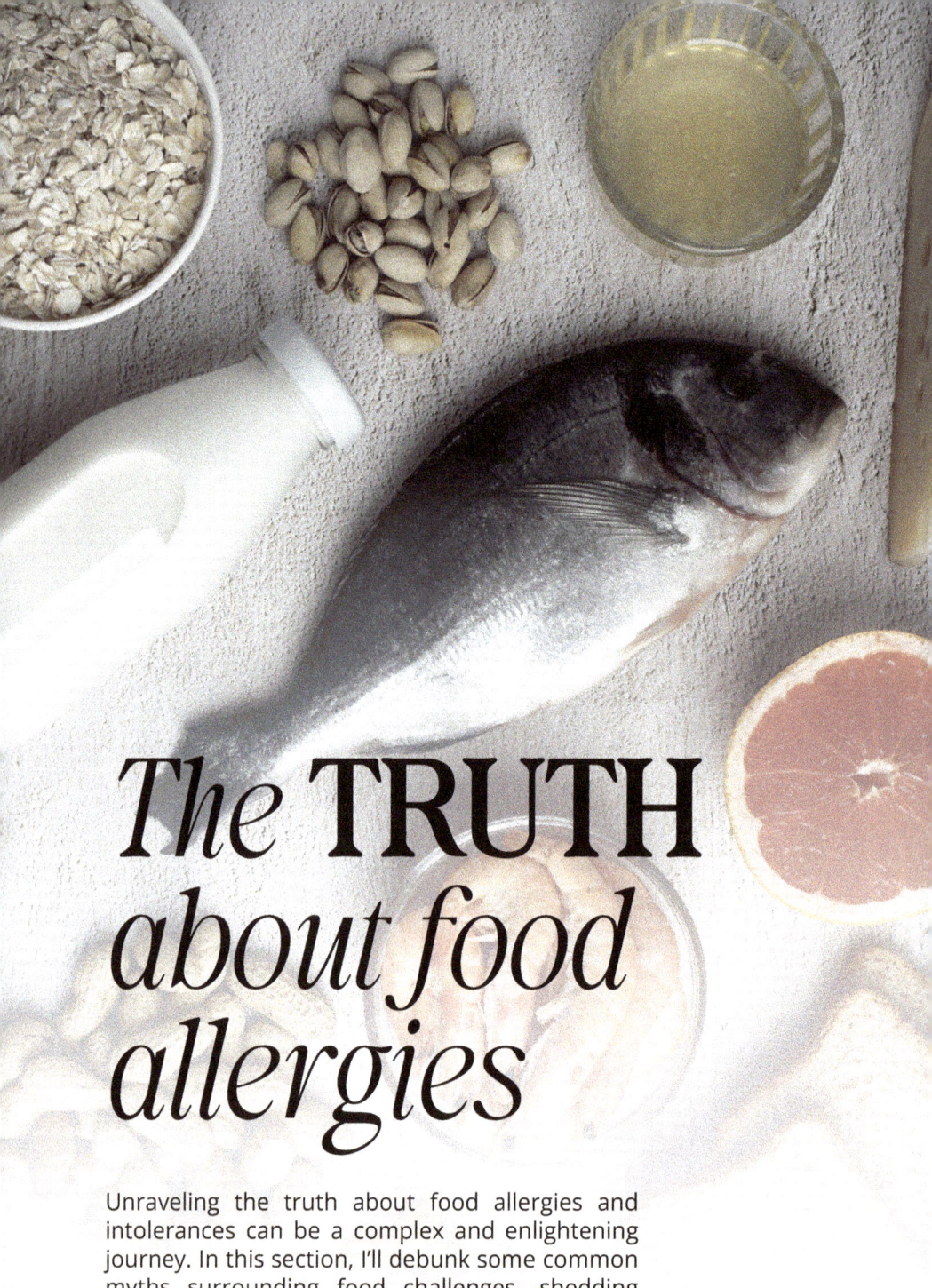

The TRUTH about food allergies

Unraveling the truth about food allergies and intolerances can be a complex and enlightening journey. In this section, I'll debunk some common myths surrounding food challenges, shedding light on the underlying realities of what many have come to believe as true.

MYTH 1

Food allergies are genetic.

Truth: While it may seem like food allergies have a genetic link, the reality is more nuanced. Infections and toxins can disrupt how our cells interact with their DNA (aka the "blueprint" of the cell), leading to altered expression that influences our responses to certain foods. For example, cilantro avoidance can be attributed to DNA changes passed through blood or other fluids from parent to child. Although it might appear genetic, it is often a consequence of unresolved infections, offering a fresh perspective on the roots of these sensitivities.

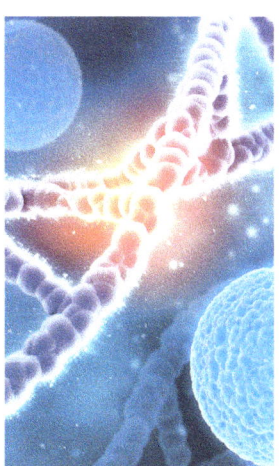

MYTH 2

Avoiding problem foods is the only solution for relief.

Truth: It's true that avoiding triggering foods can offer short-term relief, but it's not the only path to healing, and it's definitely not a lasting one. Identifying and addressing the external root cause of the symptoms is equally crucial. Avoidance can act as an initial step to reduce discomfort while we focus on improving tissue and system function. Tracking changes in food irritations can provide valuable

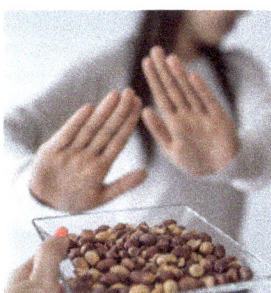

insights into progress. Once the irritant is no longer a problem, it signals that the underlying cause has been resolved, giving you the freedom to decide whether to reintroduce the food or not.

MYTH 3

It's fine not to enjoy

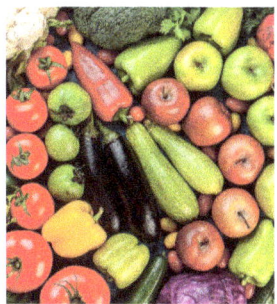

most fresh fruits and vegetables as long as you like a few.

Truth: Personal food preferences are subjective, but keep in mind that your reactions to certain foods can hold meaningful clues to your overall well-being.

Remember that avoiding fruits and vegetables due to taste or digestive issues may signify organ or system dysfunction, affecting your overall health and performance. Beyond the digestive system, these aversions could have far-reaching consequences, impacting other functions like reproductive health or mental well-being. While there's no need to consume every fruit and vegetable daily, developing a tolerance for them and occasionally incorporating a variety of fresh produce into your diet can be profoundly beneficial for your general health.

MYTH 4

Food allergies and sensitivities are a lifelong burden.

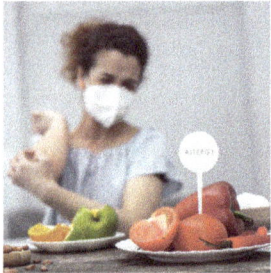

Truth: The prospect of living with food allergies indefinitely can be daunting, but there is hope. Identifying and successfully eliminating external causes can lead to a significant reduction or complete resolution of reactions to certain foods, granting a newfound sense of freedom and well-being.

MYTH 5

Many food allergies naturally fade with age.

Truth: Aging may lead to changes in hormonal levels and the gut microbiome, altering the symptoms of underlying issues, including food allergies. However, simply growing older doesn't resolve these problems. Allergies are symptoms of underlying imbalances, and without external intervention, the root causes persist. Children who experienced food allergies often grow to become teens and adults with struggle with symptoms including cystic acne, anxiety or ADHD, new seasonal allergies that didn't exist in childhood, or intense menstrual symptoms. It's crucial to address the underlying issues proactively to ensure a more profound and sustainable improvement in your overall health.

With these myths unraveled and the truth revealed, I hope you have a deeper appreciation of the multifaceted nature of food allergies and intolerances and will be able to make better-informed health choices based on your responses to certain foods.

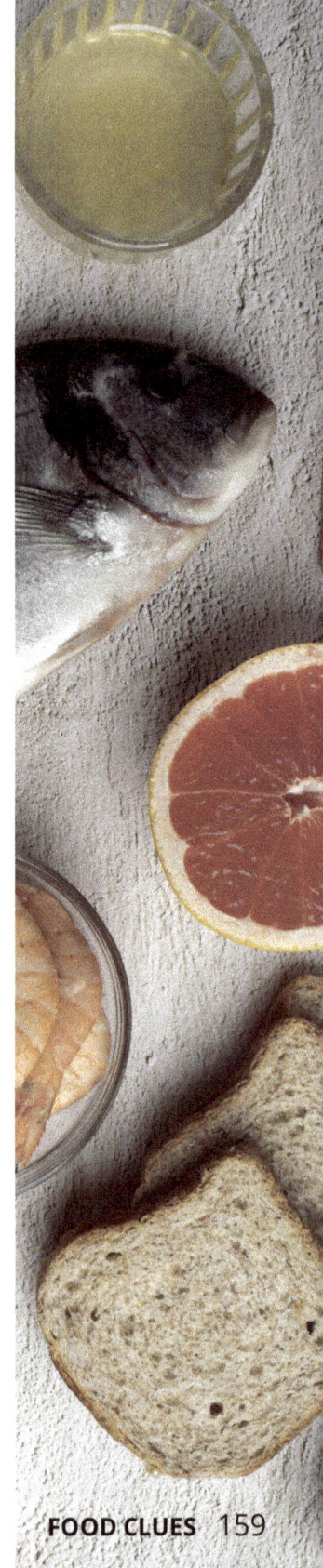

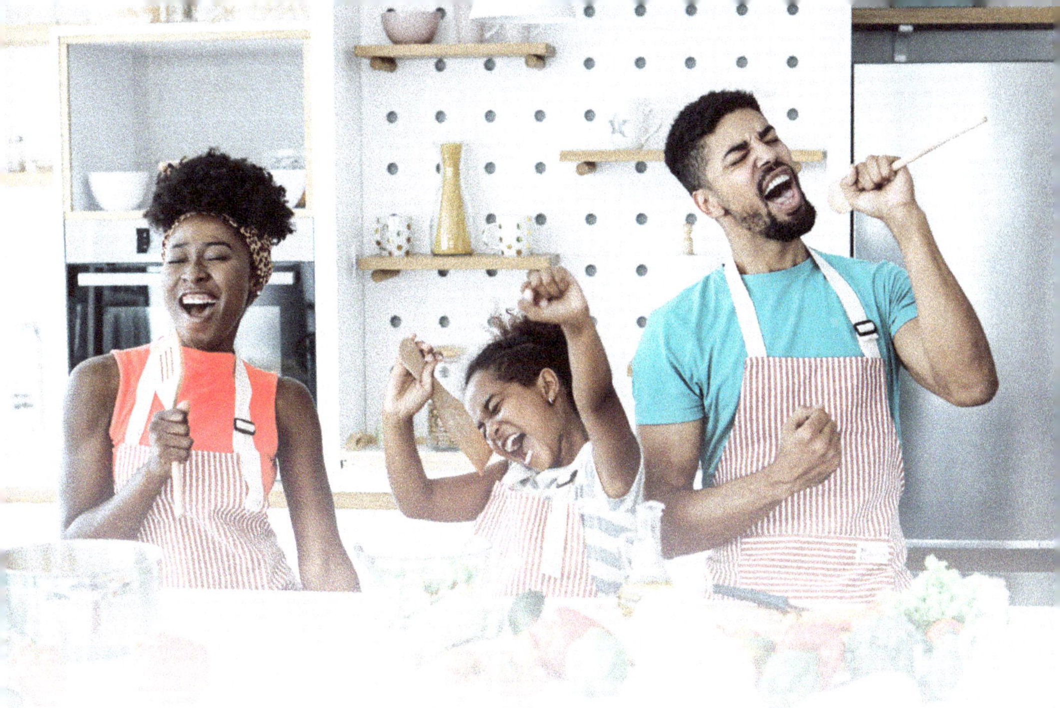

USING FOOD CLUES TO HEAL

Client success stories

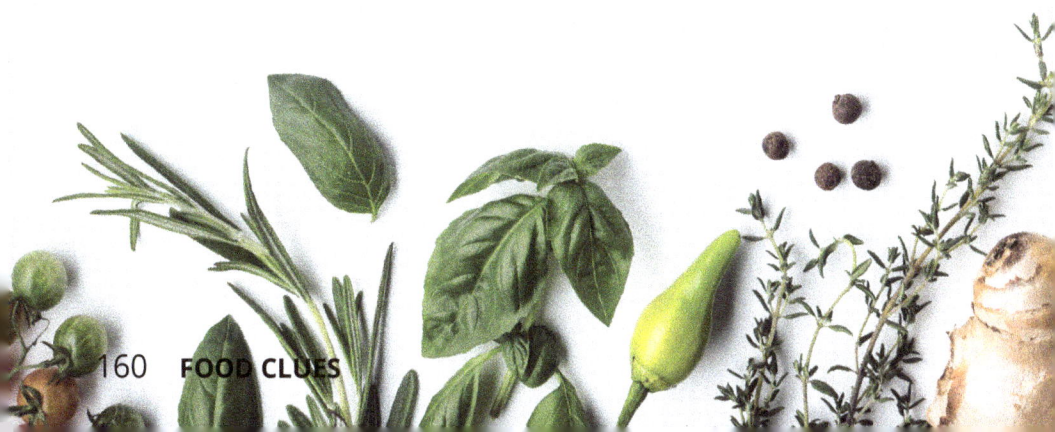

As a dedicated wellness practitioner, I have always been fascinated by the intricate connections between our bodies and the foods we consume. Over the years, my journey has been enriched by unraveling the hidden messages behind food likes and dislikes and how they serve as valuable clues to our overall health and well-being. Armed with this understanding, I have been able to create personalized treatment plans that go beyond traditional approaches, providing relief to clients suffering from chronic symptoms that seemed unresponsive to medication and conventional therapies. Let me share with you the remarkable success stories of some of my clients whose lives were transformed by identifying their food avoidances and allergies, leading us to the root causes of their health challenges.

Client 1: Peyton, 21 Years Old

Peyton, a twenty-one-year-old recent college graduate, sought help for an array of symptoms that persisted despite trying various medications. Her complaints included difficulty concentrating, persistent nausea and bloating, unrelenting headaches, and uncomfortable constipation. As I delved into her food preferences, her food clues showed that she avoided mushrooms and vinegar.

After analyzing these food clues, the pieces of the puzzle started falling into place. The avoidance of vinegar hinted at potential issues with food breakdown in the stomach, while her shunning of mushrooms suggested an elevated fungal load in the body. Her constipation and difficulty concentrating caused me to suspect that the fungal load was likely in the large intestine. Many constipation issues involve the colon (another word for a section of the large intestine), and many of the chemicals your brain uses to help with concentration and memory, like dopamine, are made in the lining of the large intestine. An increased fungal load could easily affect elimination and chemical production, causing her symptoms.

By the end of her assessment, I had successfully identified the external cause of her symptoms—a bacterial infection she contracted from her mother at birth. I suspected that the elevated fungal load was a reaction from the body to maintain proper proportions of bacterial and fungal levels in the intestines, given the presence of the bacterial infection. With this understanding, I created a treatment plan that focused on optimizing detox pathways for optimal elimination, maximizing liver performance to facilitate effective infection removal, healing the stomach and intestine, and reducing her fungal load to a safe level where additional fungi introduced to the body (like eating mushrooms) would not produce an avoidance or ill-feeling response. In eight months, Peyton's digestive symptoms were entirely resolved, her focus improved remarkably, and she even discovered a newfound ability to tolerate mushrooms, telling me that one day she was able to enjoy a delicious mushroom risotto.

Client 2: Mary, 67 years old

Mary, a vibrant and active sixty-seven-year-old, had endured twenty years of relentless nausea, frequent vomiting, abdominal discomfort, and chronic fatigue, and recently began to experience chronic bladder pain. Her efforts to find relief through conventional means had been in vain. To understand her unique challenges better, I turned to her food clues. Mary struggled with consuming red meat, gluten, and dairy. She had an aversion to vinegary foods, she had intense sugar cravings, and she admitted to often being a picky eater.

Unraveling these food clues unraveled the underlying truth—Mary's digestive system faced significant hurdles. Poor digestion and absorption, coupled with challenges in managing protein digestion and acid elimination, seemed to be at the root of her ailments.

Upon further exploration, I traced Mary's health issues back to a childhood mold infection that had never been fully addressed. After optimizing detox pathways (phase one of the Renatrition Healing Framework), we flushed her system of the mold infection and focused targeted support on healing and restoring the proper function of her digestive system.

Mary's treatment plan included visits about once a month. In less than twelve months, her energy levels rebounded, and she found herself able to enjoy all foods without the debilitating symptoms that had plagued her for over two decades.

Client 3: Judy, 60 years old

Judy, a determined sixty-year-old, was grappling with persistent pain and weakness in her left hip, causing difficulty with basic movements and positions. She walked with a limp, which was often painful, and it was often difficult to sit evenly because her left hip would rest slightly higher than her right, causing her left heel to stay off the floor. Her limp and heel position created balance challenges in sitting, standing, and walking, even causing her to use a shower chair for bathing to reduce her risk for falls. Despite previous attempts with medication and physical therapy, her symptoms persisted. In search of the underlying cause, I turned my attention to Judy's food clues. She had a shrimp allergy and gluten sensitivity and avoided coconut.

Unraveling these food clues led to a revealing conclusion, Judy's symptoms were indicative of a bacterial overload within her body. I dug deeper into her medical history and discovered a link between her condition and three external causes—a past parasitic infection, multiple surgeries, and a prior concussion. All of these findings likely contributed to reduced fluid flow and nutrient supply through the body, tightening of tissues, and the development of weakness and stiffness throughout the entire left leg.

In addition to Judy's supplement program based on the Renatrition Healing Framework to eliminate the bacteria and parasite, I incorporated intermittent strengthening and conditioning exercises for her left leg. Six months after starting her healing program, she sent me a message saying she was able to put her left heel fully on the ground while seated in her shower chair for the first time in sixteen years. She gained new confidence in her safety and movement ability.

Client 4: Macie, 13 years old

Macie's persistent back pain following scoliosis surgery was a puzzling concern for her and her family. Despite the surgery intended to alleviate her discomfort, she found herself unable to return to dance due to ongoing pain and weakness. Exploring her food clues, we discovered that she avoided hard-boiled eggs, coconut, spicy and vinegary foods, blue cheese, and mushrooms. These patterns pointed to issues with protein digestion, likely due to low stomach and intestinal lining integrity and an elevated fungal load.

Further investigation revealed a mold infection as the external root cause for her symptoms. (Side note: In nearly every client who works with me who has a diagnosis of scoliosis, I find an external cause of infection that significantly impacts liver performance. I believe this causes the liver to swell and the muscles around the liver to tighten and not move as freely, forcing a curvature in the spine that does not resolve with exercise, and symptoms that don't resolve even after surgery. This is a classic demonstration of the hierarchy of dysfunction, where the symptoms are felt near the top of the pyramid, in the muscle, but the source of the problem is actually near the bottom of the pyramid, in the gut.)

To address this, Macie's treatment approach focused on clearing detox pathways, optimizing liver performance, and reducing inflammation, and heavily focused on improving liver function. I also incorporated dance-specific strengthening and conditioning exercises for her back and hips.

Six months after starting her Renatrition program, she not only returned to dance without restrictions but also made it onto the dance competition team. Her joy and excitement were undeniable, as she was finally able to embrace her passion and return to doing what she loved.

Macie's mother was so thrilled and impressed with Macie's outcomes with her Renatrition program that she promptly enrolled her mother, son, and aunt, as well as herself, in treatment programs.

Client 5: Gil, 50 years old

Gil's journey to reclaim his health had been riddled with persistent and worsening sinus congestion along with relentless allergy symptoms that weren't responding to conventional medication. His neck, face, and belly were constantly swollen and uncomfortable, and he frequently experienced nausea after eating. A diagnosis of celiac disease, coupled with hives, eczema, and abdominal cramping, left him searching for answers. As I delved into Gil's food clues, I discovered that he had a seafood allergy and an aversion to blue cheese, mushrooms, garlic, onions, hard-boiled eggs, and spicy and vinegary foods.

I quickly concluded that Gil likely had poor protein digestion and compromised stomach and intestinal integrity, which affects nutrient absorption. It seemed that his intestines were harboring a bacterial buildup due to undigested proteins that had accumulated over time. It was entirely possible that the undigested proteins may have included high levels of gluten, resulting in his diagnosis of celiac disease.

Upon further examination, an external cause became evident—a mold infection, signified by a penicillin allergy discovered during childhood. Penicillin drugs are derived from mold spores, providing a clear indication of the underlying issue.

Gil was filled with excitement and a newfound understanding of the root causes of his health challenges. Words can't explain the relief he felt by just knowing where his symptoms were coming from, and especially why his previous efforts weren't helping. Within the first two weeks of his Renatrition program, his swelling and abdominal tenderness reduced, and he was able breathe through his nose for the first time in years.

....

These client success stories exemplify the power of understanding and using food clues to achieve true healing. By decoding the hidden messages behind their food likes and dislikes, I was able to uncover the external causes of my clients' chronic symptoms and create treatment plans tailored to their individual needs so they can live more fulfilling and active lives with fewer symptoms, increased strength and mobility, and more confidence in their ability to tolerate their daily activities. Using a combination of holistic approaches and a deep appreciation for the intricate balance between food and well-being, we experienced transformative healing journeys that not only alleviated symptoms but also improved daily physical function. These stories serve as inspiring testaments to the remarkable potential of embracing food clues as a gateway to a healthier and happier life.

It is important to highlight that while the client success stories share a common pattern of system focus and intervention, each individual's treatment plan was uniquely tailored based on their specific external causes. While we have provided an account of their healing journeys, the specific essential oils and supplements used have been intentionally omitted to protect you, the reader.

I want to emphasize that the use of exercise, essential oils, and supplements for treatment should always be conducted under the expert guidance of a qualified wellness professional. Every person's health profile and needs are distinct, and what worked effectively for one client may not yield the same results for another. In some cases, utilizing interventions without professional supervision could even impede your healing process.

Each client's success was the outcome of meticulous assessment, careful analysis, and personalized treatment based on their unique circumstances. Even though many of the intervention categories were similar—vitamins, minerals, herbal supplements, essential oils, fluid flow exercises, muscle strengthening, etc.—their dosages and delivery methods were completely different and often changed throughout their program. For example, some supplements only required one dose, while others were used for weeks. Some essential oils were rubbed topically, and some were inhaled using aromatherapy. Seeking guidance from a qualified wellness practitioner is crucial in navigating the complexities of your health journey and ensuring that your treatment plan is optimized to suit your specific needs.

As you read these inspiring stories, I hope you draw inspiration from the profound transformations that can be achieved through a holistic approach to health and wellness. But remember, there is no one-size-fits-all solution in this journey, and partnering with a qualified professional is the key to unlocking your own path to healing and well-being.

FAQs
Frequently Asked Questions

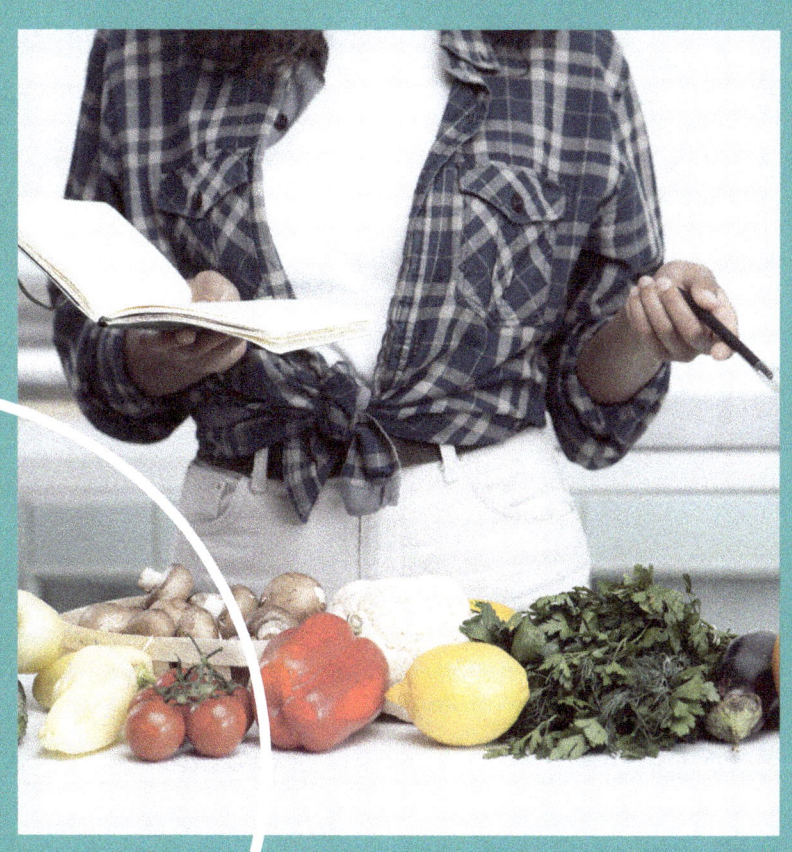

What if I'm craving some of the foods on the avoidance list? Or what if I strongly dislike a food in the craving section? Or what if my food isn't even in this book?

As I mentioned in the introduction, I selected the more common foods people avoid and crave based on my general observations and my experiences working with my clients. This book is definitely not an exclusive list of foods. Anyone can have an allergy, avoidance reaction, or craving for any food at any time. I hope to convey the message that those responses aren't merely coincidental; they have meaning. And this book provides insight into those meanings.

Here are a few tips to get you started if you have a question about a food or a food response that isn't specifically discussed in the book:

1. If you're craving a food that's generally considered to be healthy (e.g., fresh fruit, vegetable, or meat), it may indicate a nutrient deficiency or healing using a property of the food. For example, people crave eggs when their bodies need more choline due to their high natural choline content. People often crave foods like salads, carrots, and celery when they need more fiber to aid with digestion. While most of the foods in the craving section involve processing and provide little nutritional benefit, I'll highlight two items: vinegary foods and salt. Avoidance of vinegary or spicy foods could indicate an elevated acid level in the body and issues with acid elimination could be considered. Avoiding salty foods could indicate difficulty with transporting or absorbing salt, since natural salt (not basic table salt) is critical for proper cellular function.

2. Look for similar foods that are listed. For example, green beans are similar to beans and peas, reactions to most dairy products using cow's milk will be similar to the information for milk, and reactions to other leafy greens are similar to reactions to lettuce.

3. If you know your particular food is high in a certain nutrient, difficulty managing that nutrient may be the problem. Many know that carrots are high in beta carotene, which is used by the liver to make vitamin A, so avoidance of carrots could be a sign of difficulty making vitamin A. Foods like chicken, fish, or other types of meat are often high in protein; therefore, avoidance may be related to difficulty with protein digestion, similar to steak, which is included in the book

4. If you really feel stuck and can't figure out what your food clue could mean, feel free to message me at dralexissams@gmail.com, and I'll do my best to assist you.

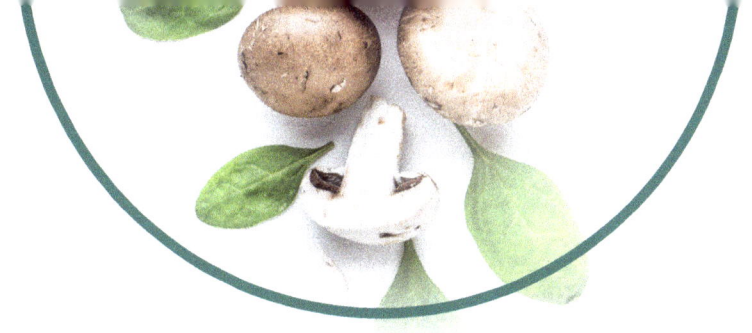

A lot of foods that I avoid are mentioned in the book. Does that mean my health is at a significant risk for something?

That's hard to say. In general, the number or intensity of signs and symptoms doesn't correlate to the stage or severity of any condition or disease. Signs and symptoms can be how your body tells you to check something because of a problem. They don't necessarily tell you where or what the problem is.

When clients have a long list of symptoms, I tell them to think about it conceptually like sound volume. One or two symptoms could be considered a whisper, especially if they don't create any pain or discomfort (e.g., skin moles). If you don't listen to the whisper, the body may try to "talk louder" by revealing more symptoms.

What if I simply don't like a food? Is that a problem?

It could be. One of the main differences between disliking a food and avoiding a food is whether symptoms are created or not. If you stay away from a food because a specific reaction occurs when you eat it, I would consider that an avoidance that is likely related to an issue in the body somewhere that may need to be addressed. This includes taste. If a food tastes bad (and it's not spoiled in any way), that is likely an avoidance as well. Food choices without strong taste aversions or other symptoms may be more related to personal preferences based on environment, culture, or other general factors.

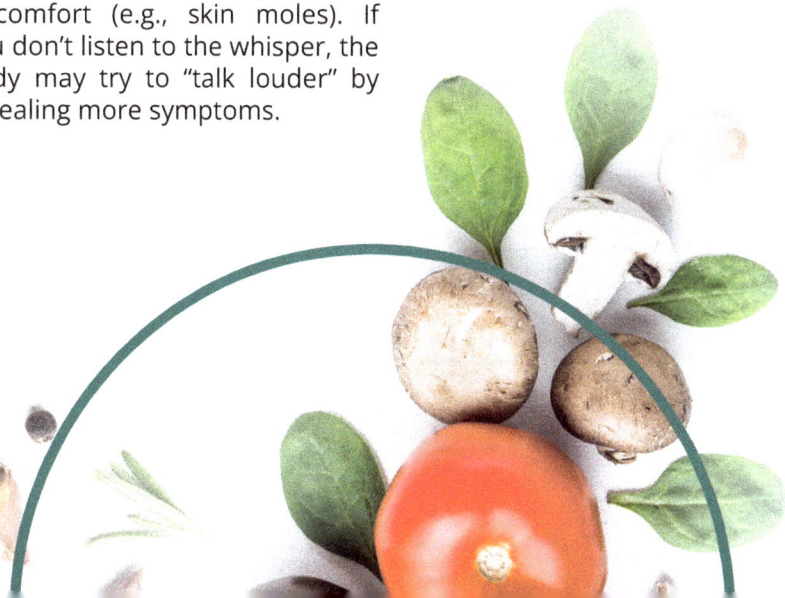

Why isn't my doctor talking about any of these things?

I am often asked this question one of two times during a client's healing experience with me: at the end of the assessment when all of their questions are answered and they have a clear picture that explains all of their symptoms, or at the end of their program when they've achieved the relief they've been searching for.

In short, it's a matter of treatment perspective. Some health professionals don't talk about certain treatment concepts because it's not their primary method of treatment.

I truly believe every health and wellness professional seeks to provide their patients and clients with the best care they can provide. That said, I also believe a practitioner's ability to treat and support the people they care for is highly related to their education and their treatment "toolbox," the additional skills and knowledge they possess to accomplish their work.

Surgeons are largely taught to use surgery as a healing tool and look for ways surgery can help their patients. Medical doctors are largely taught to focus on diseases and reducing symptoms to help their patients find relief. They may also specialize in a certain area, so their focus may relate to finding problems in a certain area or function. Dentists look for tooth issues. Dermatologists focus on the skin. Endocrinologists look for hormone issues.

In a larger context, I also believe that healthcare in the United States focuses more on reactive care for issues once they've developed into a disease or condition instead of preventative care which focuses on improving and maintaining healthy performance of organs and tissues before they become dysfunctional and cause disease.

While my education as a physical therapist was rooted in looking at the musculoskeletal system to help patients, I quickly realized that understanding the connections between all the organs and body systems was more beneficial to helping clients heal. It just made sense; all body organs and systems work together all the time in order for us to live and function. No single area ever works alone.

The thought of just focusing on one area and not looking at any others in order to treat a condition seemed shortsighted to me, so I focus on adding to my toolbox. I seek to deepen my knowledge of all body systems and functions along with treatment methods that involve natural solutions because I believe they are more easily accepted by the body with fewer side effects. Expanding my methods of treatment allows me to see signs, symptoms, and patterns that others may not, making my treatment plans more effective and efficient.

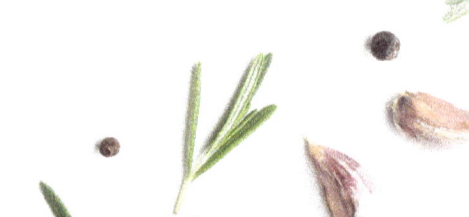

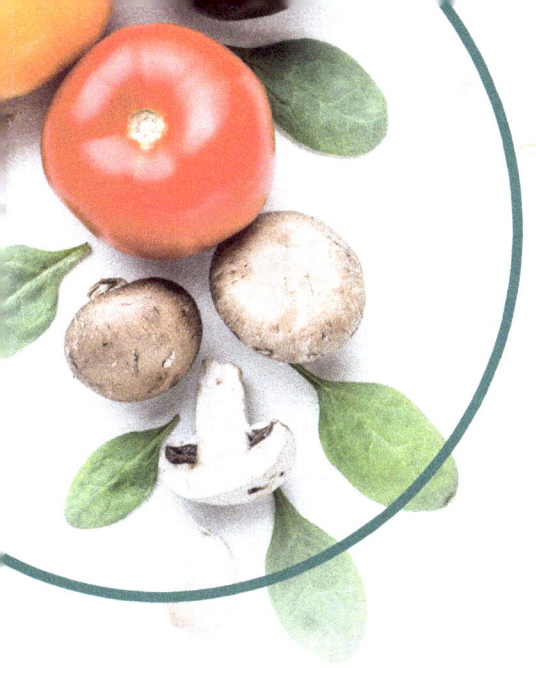

Does Renatrition accept clients from anywhere?

Yes. I work with clients out of my office in Phoenix, Arizona, but also work with clients virtually all over the world!

What do I need to do to work with Renatrition?

If you would like to schedule an assessment session with Dr. Sams, visit https://renatrition.com/assessment for more info.

What guarantee is there that a Renatrition program will work for me?

While no treatment or program from any practitioner can ever be guaranteed, what I do promise my clients are answers. I can guarantee that after a full Renatrition Assessment, you will have all of your external causes identified and an answer that explains all of your symptoms and conditions.

Could a Renatrition program help me avoid surgery?

I have been able to help numerous clients avoid surgery once their external causes have been identified and resolved. Surgeries often involve the removal of a failing organ or repair of an injured area but don't always consider the cause of the failure or injury. By addressing those through a Renatrition program, you could avoid surgery and support the problem areas to heal and return to normal function.

Could a Renatrition program help me get off of my prescription meds?

Similar to surgery, many prescriptions focus on reducing a symptom or improving organ function without addressing the cause of dysfunction. Doing so with a Renatrition program has allowed my clients to work with their doctors and successfully wean off of numerous prescription medications, including artificial insulin, thyroid medication, antidepressants, and medications for attention deficit disorder.

About Dr. Alexis

Dr. Alexis Sams, PT, NKT, is one of the most successful practitioners of functional medicine and holistic health care.

As the founder of Renatrition Health & Wellness, she has worked with hundreds of clients and companies all over the world, focusing on using a unique treatment approach that uses food choices and preferences to find things that often go overlooked in more traditional medical practice. Her treatment programs have helped those who couldn't get a clear answer for the cause of their condition or symptoms, especially when exercises, medications, injections, or surgery did not work.

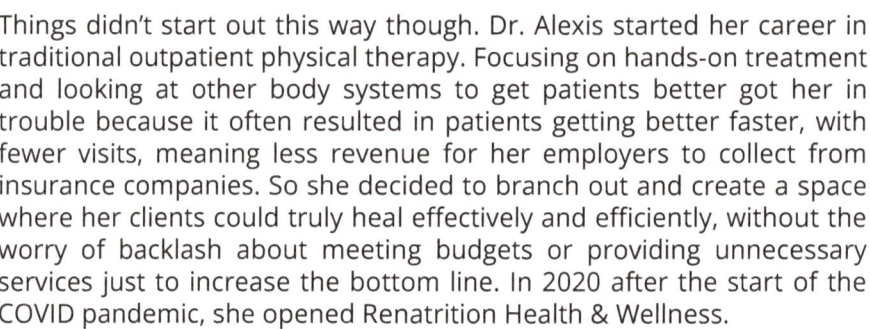

Things didn't start out this way though. Dr. Alexis started her career in traditional outpatient physical therapy. Focusing on hands-on treatment and looking at other body systems to get patients better got her in trouble because it often resulted in patients getting better faster, with fewer visits, meaning less revenue for her employers to collect from insurance companies. So she decided to branch out and create a space where her clients could truly heal effectively and efficiently, without the worry of backlash about meeting budgets or providing unnecessary services just to increase the bottom line. In 2020 after the start of the COVID pandemic, she opened Renatrition Health & Wellness.

Today, Dr. Alexis runs a thriving clinic based in Phoenix, Arizona, and continues to work with clients worldwide. She is committed to providing quality care with natural, non-surgical, and non-prescription solutions and fully resolving the causes that hold clients back from feeling and performing at their best, combining her extensive training in physical therapy, functional medicine, mindset coaching, and herbalism.

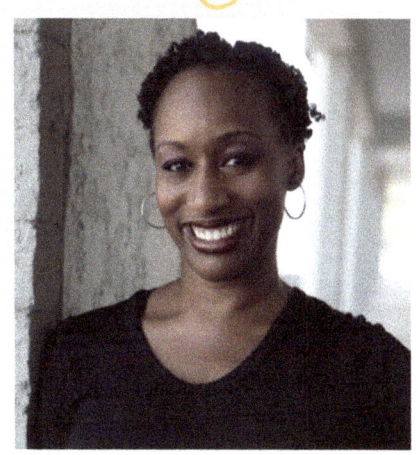

FOOD Clues

Dr. Alexis Sams, PT
The Food Allergy Doc

 renatrition.com/links

 renatrition.com/blog

 dralexissams@gmail.com

 603-730-4159

 SPREAKING AND EVENTS
renatrition.com/dralexis

https://renatrition.com/foodallergytotalfreedomprogram

INFO AND MEDIA

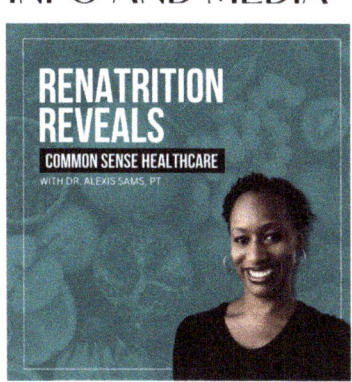

PODCAST

 Renatrition Reveals

 Renatrition Reveals

SOCIAL MEDIA

 The Food Allergy Freedom Collective: Treatment Solutions Beyond Avoidance

 @dralexissams

 @renatrition

 @dralexissams

 Dr. Alexis Sams

Gain immediate access to live links, updates, and more!

SCAN FOR LINKS!

FOOD ALLERGY
Freedom Collective

Read Client Stories, Ask Questions, and Learn About Treatment Solutions Beyond Just Avoiding Foods!

SCAN TO JOIN OUR FACEBOOK COMMUNITY

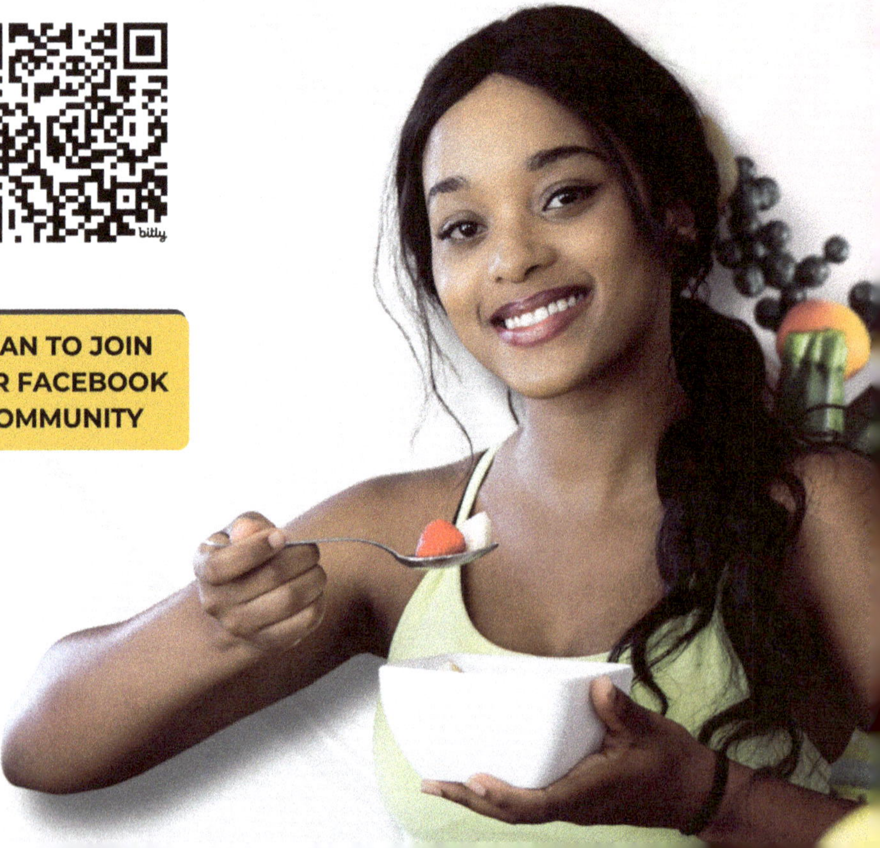

Acknowledgements

I would like to express my deepest gratitude to the incredible individuals who have played a vital role in the creation of this book, Food Clues: Decoding the Hidden Messages Behind Your Food Likes and Dislikes. Their unwavering support, invaluable insights, and endless inspiration have been instrumental in bringing this project to fruition.

First and foremost, I would like to thank some special clients whose dedication to the process of true healing sparked the initial inspiration for this book: Jamie, Macie, Judy, Mary, Ronda, Payton, Kacey, Red, and Ashleigh. Your commitment to the program and to understanding the intricate relationship between food and health planted the seeds that grew into this transformative work.

I extend my heartfelt appreciation to TaVona, whose unwavering support and belief in this project kept me motivated during moments of self-doubt. Your encouragement and words of wisdom provided the necessary fuel to persevere and overcome the challenges that came my way.

To my parents, Melvena, Phillip, and Bruce, thank you for your unwavering love and understanding. Your patience and encouragement sustained me through the long hours of research and writing. Your belief in me and this project is a constant source of inspiration.

To Adriano, your unwavering support and belief in my work have been a constant source of inspiration. Your firsthand experience with the transformative power of using food clues to improve health has enriched the essence of this book, and I am forever grateful for your love and encouragement.

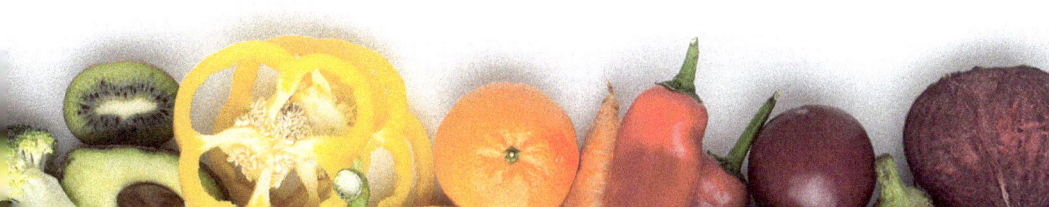

· ·

To my remarkable work partner and cherished friend, Lisa, your invaluable contribution to this book goes beyond measure. Your exceptional organizational skills and keen insights helped shape the sections and fill the missing gaps, elevating the entire project to its fullest potential. Through the challenges and triumphs, you stood by my side, keeping our shared vision afloat, and I am deeply grateful for your unwavering support. This book is a testament to our enduring partnership and friendship, and I couldn't have done it without you.

To my editor, Stacey, thank you for your meticulous attention to detail and invaluable editorial guidance. Your keen eye and insightful suggestions have elevated the quality of this book and polished its message.

Lastly, but certainly not least, I would like to express my heartfelt gratitude to the readers of this book. Your curiosity, open-mindedness, and willingness to explore the depths of the intricate relationship between food and health are the ultimate driving force behind this work. It is my sincere hope that Food Clues empowers you to embark on a transformative journey toward optimal health and well-being.

This book was written for each and every one of you. Your support, guidance, and inspiration have shaped its very essence. May our collective efforts continue to shed light on the hidden messages behind our food likes and dislikes, and may they pave the way for a healthier and more vibrant future.

With heartfelt appreciation,

Alexis

· ·

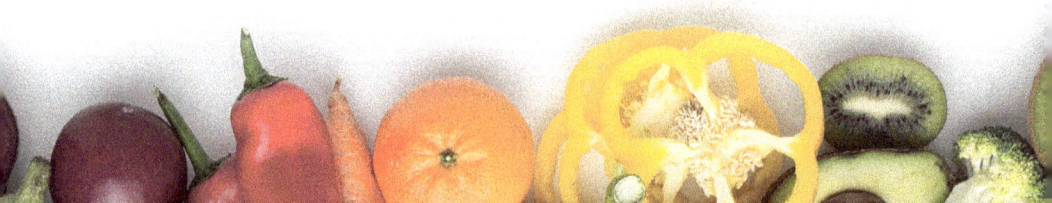

References

ACAAI. "Egg." *ACAAI Patient,* 21 Mar. 2019, acaai.org/allergies/allergic-conditions/food/egg/.

Alonso, Leonardo L., et al. "Shellfish Allergy." *PubMed,* StatPearls Publishing, 2023, www.ncbi.nlm.nih.gov/books/NBK448089/#:~:text=Shellfish%20%20allergies%20can%20occur%20due. Accessed 2 Dec. 2023.

Arya, Shalini S., et al. "Peanuts as Functional Food: A Review." *Journal of Food Science and Technology,* vol. 53, no. 1, 19 Sept. 2015, pp. 31–41, www.ncbi.nlm.nih.gov/pmc/articles/PMC4711439/, https://doi.org/10.1007/s13197-015-2007-9. Accessed 24 Feb. 2019.

Boquien, Clair-Yves. "Human Milk: An Ideal Food for Nutrition of Preterm Newborn."
Frontiers in Pediatrics, vol. 6, 16 Oct. 2018, www.frontiersin.org/articles/10.3389/fped.2018.00295/full, https://doi.org/10.3389/fped.2018.00295.

Czaja-Bulsa, Grażyna, and Michał Bulsa. "What Do We Know Now about IgE-Mediated Wheat Allergy in Children?" *Nutrients,* vol. 9, no. 1, 4 Jan. 2017, p. 35, https://doi.org/10.3390/nu9010035. Accessed 16 Mar. 2019.

Elisabetta Del Duca, et al. "Fatty-Acid-Based Membrane Lipidome Profile of Peanut Allergy Patients: An Exploratory Study of a Lifelong Health Condition." *International Journal of Molecular Sciences,* vol. 24, no. 1, 21 Dec. 2022, pp. 120–120,
https://doi.org/10.3390/ijms24010120. Accessed 6 Sept. 2023.

Elli, Luca, et al. "Diagnosis of Gluten Related Disorders: Celiac Disease, Wheat Allergy and Non-Celiac Gluten Sensitivity." *World Journal of Gastroenterology,* vol. 21, no. 23, 21
June 2015, pp. 7110–7119, https://doi.org/10.3748/wjg.v21.i23.7110.

"Food Allergy & Anaphylaxis Connection Team | Food Allergy & Anaphylaxis." *www.foodallergyawareness.org,* www.foodallergyawareness.org/food-allergy-and-anaphylaxis/foodallergens/fish/. Accessed 2 Dec. 2023.

Gupta, R. S., et al. "The Prevalence, Severity, and Distribution of Childhood Food Allergy in the United States." *PEDIATRICS,* vol. 128, no. 1, 20 June 2011, pp. e9–e17,
https://doi.org/10.1542/peds.2011-0204.

Kong, J., et al. "Comprehensive Metabolomics Identifies the Alarmin Uric Acid as a Critical Signal for the Induction of Peanut Allergy." *Allergy,* vol. 70, no. 5, 2 Mar. 2015, pp.

495–505, https://doi.org/10.1111/all.12579. Accessed 2 Apr. 2022.

Lack, Gideon, et al. "Factors Associated with the Development of Peanut Allergy in Childhood." *The New England Journal of Medicine,* vol. 348, no. 11, 13 Mar. 2003, pp. 977–985, ncbi.nlm.nih.gov/pubmed/12637607, https://doi.org/10.1056/NEJMoa013536.

Reber, Laurent L., et al. "The Pathophysiology of Anaphylaxis." *Journal of Allergy and Clinical Immunology,* vol. 140, no. 2, 2018, pp. 335–348, www.ncbi.nlm.nih.gov/pmc/articles/PMC5657389/, https://doi.org/10.1016/j.jaci.2017.06.003.

Sicherer, Scott H, et al. "US Prevalence of Self-Reported Peanut, Tree Nut, and Sesame Allergy: 11-Year Follow-Up." *The Journal of Allergy and Clinical Immunology,* vol. 125, no. 6, 2010, pp. 1322–6, www.ncbi.nlm.nih.gov/pubmed/20462634, https://doi.org/10.1016/j.jaci.2010.03.029.

Sicherer, Scott H., et al. "Prevalence of Peanut and Tree Nut Allergy in the US Determined by a Random Digit Dial Telephone Survey." *Journal of Allergy and Clinical Immunology,* vol. 103, no. 4, Apr. 1999, pp. 559–562, https://doi.org/10.1016/s0091-6749(99)70224-1. Accessed 1 Nov. 2020.

Simopoulos, A. P. "Evolutionary Aspects of Diet and Essential Fatty Acids." *World Review of Nutrition and Dietetics,* vol. 88, 2001, pp. 18–27, pubmed.ncbi.nlm.nih.gov/11935953/.
https://doi.org/10.1159/000059742. Accessed 2 Dec. 2023.

Simopoulos, Artemis P. "The Importance of the Omega-6/Omega-3 Fatty Acid Ratio in Cardiovascular Disease and Other Chronic Diseases." *Experimental Biology and Medicine (Maywood, N.J.),* vol. 233, no. 6, 2008, pp. 674–88, www.ncbi.nlm.nih.gov/pubmed/18408140, https://doi.org/10.3181/0711-MR-311.

Storhaug, Christian Løvold, et al. "Country, Regional, and Global Estimates for Lactose Malabsorption in Adults: A Systematic Review and Meta-Analysis." *The Lancet Gastroenterology & Hepatology,* vol. 2, no. 10, Oct. 2017, pp. 738–746,
www.thelancet.com/journals/langas/article/PIIS2468-1253(17)30154-1/fulltext,
https://doi.org/10.1016/s2468-1253(17)30154-1.

Warren, Christopher M., et al. "Prevalence and Severity of Sesame Allergy in the United States." *JAMA Network Open,* vol. 2, no. 8, 2 Aug. 2019, p. e199144, https://doi.org/10.1001/jamanetworkopen.2019.9144. Accessed 16 Dec. 2019.

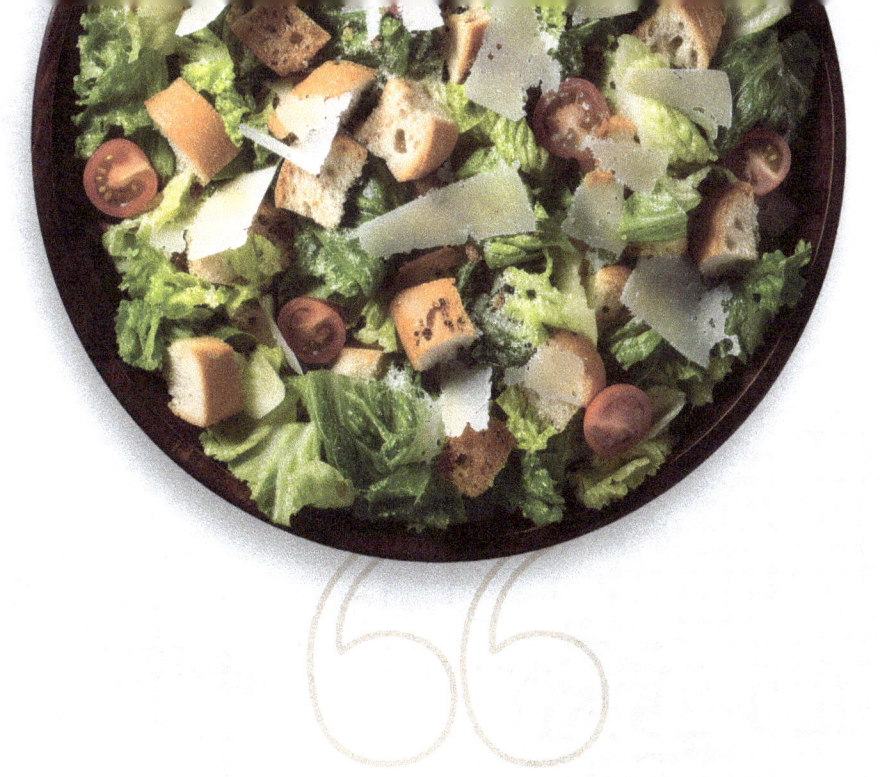

FREEDOM
from food allergies and intolerances
IS POSSIBLE.

www.ingramcontent.com/pod-product-compliance
Lightning Source LLC
Chambersburg PA
CBHW052030030426
42337CB00027B/4939